# Why Things Hurt

# Praise for *Why Things Hurt*

'First and foremost, *Why Things Hurt* is a great read. Through his interaction with thousands of patients, Brent has developed a unique and special insight into how our bodies work, both on a functional and holistic level. What is remarkable is how he has translated this into a book that has useful lessons and guidance for everyone; there is valuable learning here in terms of how to manage pain, both physically and psychologically, as well as how to prevent it. He advocates for a multidisciplinary approach to pain management which is key. A must read, even if you don't hurt, yet.'

–Dr. Kenneth Ryan, *MD, Anesthesiologist*

"Brent Stevenson is at the vanguard of manual therapy, in positioning our internal organ anatomy as integral, not peripheral, to movement patterns and musculoskeletal pain resolution. An engaging little book!"

–Annabel Mackenzie, *Shiatsu Therapist & Barral Institute Instructor*

"*Why Things Hurt* takes you on a wildly entertaining journey of discovery into how your body actually works or doesn't work, and how to fix it according to Brent's unique mastery of physiotherapy, IMS, and complex problem solving. Being a detail-oriented PhD scientist, and having competed at numerous world championships in triathlon and mountain running, this book is a fantastic resource for keeping my body moving and pain-free even with all the twists and turns life throws at me!

–Mike McMillan, *PhD Scientist & Triathlete*

"Brent Stevenson has the unique combination of being an excellent therapist and amazing teacher. In this book he has delivered some of the more complex and layered concepts in a very digestible format. This book is equally beneficial for the client as well as the practitioner."

–Harry Toor, *Physiotherapist & Illustrator*

**Why Things Hurt**
Life Lessons from an Injury-prone Physical Therapist
by Brent Stevenson, MScPT, BHKin, RCAMT, CGIMS

Sections of this book first appeared on the author's website, www.whythingshurt.com

For general information or questions, please visit www.whythingshurt.com

ISBN-13: 978-0-9953241-1-4 (electronic version)

ISBN-13: 978-0-9953241-0-7 (print version)

Published by Brent Stevenson Physiotherapy Corp.
Printed in the United States of America
Editors: Meagan Dyer, Laura Galloway
Illustrator: Harry Toor
Graphic Designer: Laura Galloway
Photography (front and back cover): Kevin Clark

# Why Things Hurt

## LIFE LESSONS FROM AN
## INJURY-PRONE PHYSICAL THERAPIST

### BRENT STEVENSON MScPT, BHKin, RCAMT, CGIMS

whythingshurt.com

To my wife and mother:
thank you and sorry for having to endure all my
unintended research. I'll try to be good, I promise.

# Contents

Myths to Dispel:
- Time heals all wounds
- Chronic pain has one root cause
- You didn't do anything wrong

# Why and How You Should Read This Book

*Why Things Hurt* is about creating a context for what it means to live healthy and pain free, both mentally and physically. I have written this book based on my experiences as an injury-prone athlete, a father, and a physiotherapist who has had the opportunity to work closely with some of the world's best healers. As I guide you through my journeys of being both the patient and the practitioner, you will begin to develop a framework for understanding where common and unusual pains originate. I have grown used to my long, lanky, loose-jointed body, and along the way I have learned a great deal about posture, pain, movement, doctors, and medical systems. *Why Things Hurt* is my way of sharing with you the points which I believe are important about how your body and your mind work as you navigate through your own journey.

Many of you want to exercise and be healthy, but perhaps you don't know how or are too scared to try because you don't want to hurt yourself. Others are trying hard every day but may be armed with poor or misleading information about what you should be doing to help yourself. For those who are too afraid to get moving, this book will help create peace of mind and a platform to begin, and it may challenge the direction and mindset of those already working on their bodies.

I have not provided charts and numbers with specific programs that I think will help everyone, but instead have focused on developing principles to follow and lessons that I think everyone should learn. Many of the principles in this book require videos to fully understand, so I have developed a series of video playlists that are integrated into the written posts on my website WhyThingsHurt.com. Different people learn in different ways, so I encourage you to read, watch, and do throughout this book. I discuss a wide range of topics, including posture, feet, shoes, sports, pregnancy, intramuscular stimulation (IMS) dry needling, osteopathy, mental health, and medical systems, which are broken into digestible articles. These articles should be comprehensible and informative to any person interested in learning about how their body works.

# Introduction:
# Getting to Know Brent

Everyone is his or her own brand of crazy. If you think you are normal, you probably don't experience a broad-enough sample of people on a daily basis. I am a physiotherapist who sees a new person every half hour for most of the day, and if I didn't appreciate the crazy in everyone, my job would drive me nuts. Thankfully, because I learn from my work every day, I love what I do. I am fascinated by how people arrive at their current physical and mental state, and that their perspective of the world is based on what they judge to be "normal."

I have the opportunity to see who people really are more than most, because clients come into my life in a vulnerable position and are asking for help. People meet me usually knowing that they have some sort of problem that they need help resolving, but they don't really have any idea of how I might help them; their friend just said, "Go see this guy, he helped me." I enter some people's lives as their primary contact with a healthcare professional, and others as their proclaimed "last hope" after having already "tried everything." The patient's physical and emotional confidence are on display to a relative stranger, so I have to be careful to try and engage with my clients in a way that places their confidence in me, based on my reading of their level of unique craziness.

My day becomes comparable to nine hours of speed dating mixed with problem solving, detective work, and cognitive behavioral therapy. I treat CEOs, nurses, entrepreneurs, MMA fighters, eighty-five-year-olds, pole dancers and construction workers, so I learn new things each day about different worlds from very unique perspectives. Gaining an appreciation of what others do all day grounds you as a person.

While I am getting to know my clients, I am charged with the task of solving their three-dimensional, moving-puzzle-of-a-pain problem. I must understand their emotional needs of how they are dealing with the pain, create a working model of what I think is causing it, and explain it to them in layman's terms in effort to move forward.

I spent a few years working almost exclusively with golfers, and I was sent to Philadelphia for a week of training as part of my job. I learned a lot about golf, but my biggest take-away was learning how to deal with wealthy, stubborn, aging men and their bodies. I was twenty-five years old, had been a physiotherapist for only one year, and found myself in a room with fifty-year-old CEOs for three hours while I assessed their bodies from head to toe, including video analysis. I then had to pitch to them a six-month plan of one-on-one sessions that would end up costing around $3,000. I learned a lot about what makes people tick. I learned to speak golf lingo and, more importantly, how to explain an "old guy's" back problem in the context of his golf swing—a task meaningful to him. When I showed these men how I could help them hit a golf ball thirty yards further by making their body move better, the fact that their pain would go away was almost secondary, and they would ask, "Where do I sign?"

I ended up leaving that position two weeks before my wedding and immediately began a few different locum positions over the summer. It was a big eye-opener of how physiotherapy clinics can differ so broadly in their models of practice. I understood that I was in a fairly unique sport-performance business before, but what I stepped into next changed the path of my career. I started working three days a week at a very busy run-down clinic in a poor, multicultural neighborhood that had me seeing four to six people per hour. I also started working two days a week at a nicer, very busy clinic in a wealthy part of town, where I would see three to four clients per hour. Both had me hooking people up to machines, juggling multiple clients at once in small curtained-off areas of a big open room. I was making good money, but started questioning whether this was what I wanted to do with my life.

In 2006—three years into my career as a physiotherapist—I decided to start my own business. I had been involved with a few clinics that were poorly run, but managed to do pretty well, so I figured, if they can do it then why can't I? I found a new personal training center that was just opening up and had two private rooms that opened onto the gym floor. The owners were looking to rent them out to a chiropractor, but I sold them on the idea of physiotherapy being better suited for the space. I had selected a name—Envision Physiotherapy—and was just about to get started when I received an email from Diane Lee, a world-respected physiotherapist and educator with a clinic about an hour away from where I lived. She was offering me a job.

I had just committed to starting a business, ten minutes from my house in the center of Vancouver, so initially I turned down the option of working an hour away from home with a world-class mentor. It took me two weeks to reconsider. I decided that, at three years into my career, I needed a mentor and that I was going to try and have both. I took the job and started working half-days in White Rock and half-days in Vancouver, trying to build a caseload in two cities at once. Diane's clinic challenged me as a physiotherapist and taught me how to build a classy, effective clinic that is both a good work environment for therapists and a positive healing environment for clients. I was back in my comfort zone of having no electrical modalities and at least thirty minutes of one-on-one time with each client. The challenge was that I had an entirely new type of clientele with which to work. Diane is best known for her work on the pelvis, and as a result we noticed a relative skew toward women's health issues. We also seemed to attract people who had already seen physiotherapists, chiropractors, and massage therapists, and had heard that our clinic could provide something different.

I tried to be a sponge around Diane and take in all the knowledge and experience I could, because I knew I wasn't going to be there forever and I wanted to push the envelope in my own way, but I still needed to gain more tools and experience. Diane's clinic exposed me to a number of good therapists, many of whom used a technique called intramuscular stimulation, or IMS, a skill that would later change the path of my career again.

I gained experience in White Rock working with women, clients with chronic pain, and seniors for half of the day, and then I drove back to Vancouver where I worked alongside personal trainers for the other half. I learned about movement and strength training from some of those trainers, and from simply having the opportunity to observe what happens in a fitness facility all day. I did countless free screening consults for new gym members and developed a new appreciation for people's fitness goals, as well as their lack of understanding of their own bodies. I networked with massage therapists, Pilates instructors, and a few key doctors, including one physician whom I had been treating since my days at the golf business.

While my learning curve at Diane's clinic was plateauing, my business in Vancouver was growing. The biggest setback for Envision Physiotherapy was my only being present half of the time, so I decided to take the leap and be fully self-employed just a few months before my wife would give birth to our first child.

Throughout all of this, I had been taking what seemed like countless post-graduate courses in attempt to develop my skills and put more tools in my toolbox as a physical therapist. Each course proved helpful, but in 2008 when I was certified by Dr. Chan Gunn, from the Institute for the Study and Treatment of Pain (iSTOP), to utilize IMS, it felt like someone had just given me a superpower, making me question what I had been doing up to that point. The effects of this "dry needling" technique were so profound that it almost seemed to work like magic. I was fixing problems that others couldn't fix— and quickly. My caseload of clients grew rapidly by word-of-mouth referrals, with people coming in saying, "I want what she had." I organically started using IMS more and more because it just worked, and clients recognized that.

The IMS certification came at a junction in my life where I took my first break from structured education and shifted into the life lessons of parenting. I had gone straight from high school, to completing my undergraduate degree in human kinetics, and then directly into a Master of Science in Physiotherapy. For the first five years of my career I was constantly taking weekend courses or undertaking some form of training, but after IMS certification and the birth of our first child, I stopped to synthesize what I had learned. I started approaching issues in my way and learning more from myself instead of others. It was an important time in my career, and an exhausting yet rewarding time in my personal life. We continued growing our family, having three kids in three years, a feat I never would have never survived without my amazingly strong wife.

Once I was fully on my own at Envision Physiotherapy, I started to realize that I enjoyed the business side of operating a clinic just as much as the physiotherapy side of things. I plotted and schemed how I was going to grow. I connected with Dr Harvey, the doctor who had set me on this path in the first place. She had just moved her practice into a brand new healthcare center beside Vancouver General Hospital and had teamed up with four other physicians to form Westcoast Family Practice. The building was the largest of its kind in the province. It housed a wide range of medical disciplines as well as the UBC medical school. I tried to pitch her on a preventative health program for her clients. Her response was, "Well, I don't think that will work in this environment, but why don't you just come join us?"

I questioned how that might work given that I already had an office, but I agreed to meet with all five of the doctors together. It was me—a physiotherapist just five years into my career—pitching to five doctors, each with twenty years of experience, on the benefits of what I do. They seemed to like me, and offered me some space in their practice; I just had to figure out how to be in two places at once. This office would give my company instant credibility and connections in the medical world, so I needed to find a solution, and I found one in my now-partner and illustrator of this book, Harry Toor. Harry was a physiotherapist with whom I had crossed paths a few times over the previous year, and he seemed to be looking to branch out on his own. I brought him on to help me launch the new location and eventually as a partner in the whole business.

While on hiatus from formal education, I came to realize that I had a passion for writing and wanted it to be a bigger part of my life. I had started a blog a few years earlier—largely to figure out what blogs actually were—and I discovered that it was a great way for me to process my thoughts. I was learning from myself by organizing my ideas and writing them down in a way that was hopefully going to be helpful for my clients. I found that I was explaining concepts and showing clients exercises that were counterintuitive and quite subtle. I was routinely asked for a resource that I could direct people to so they could learn more, but what I was showing and teaching them was somewhat against the grain and not readily available on the Internet. So I decided to make the resource myself. In the very little spare time I had, I started working on my website called WhyThingsHurt.com. I wrote articles and produced basic videos to explain the concepts of movement that I was trying to convey.

This book was born out of my website because I felt it necessary to compile my articles to create a bigger picture for people while still offering them the "choose your own adventure" option on the website. Most people will research their symptoms on the Internet and create a surface knowledge about their "condition," which can be both helpful and harmful. It is valuable to educate yourself, but learning more information without developing a context of how to process it can cause unnecessary fear and sometimes lead people down the wrong path.

The purpose of my book and the website is to help create that context for people: what health is and why things really happen to us. If behavioral change is required to fix something, telling somebody what he or she has doesn't go very far—but explain why and you will see people take action to help themselves.

My writing is an ongoing process, but after a few years my interest had piqued enough to return to the formal education world. I had a busy caseload and a growing business, but my intrigue for a technique called visceral manipulation wouldn't go away. Diane Lee had exposed this to me, and I now found myself working with a massage therapist who specialized in working with people's guts. We worked well together. She understood the value of IMS for her clients, and I gained an appreciation of the role people's organs played in their pain, alignment, and general well-being. It started me down a rabbit hole of learning what is called osteopathic manual therapy—a discipline of gentle hands-on treatments based purely on anatomy, the skill of touch, and listening to the body. I am only a few years into this journey as a practitioner, but I can already tell that visceral and neural manipulation are skills that will help me fix ailments that others cannot understand.

I offer this book as a collection of stories that I have experienced, and lessons that I have learned over thirty-seven years of being a multi-sport athlete, a physiotherapist, and a father of three. I have endured countless injuries, from minor to severe. I have worked closely with some of the world's best healers and have helped thousands of clients through various levels of pain, disability, and despair. I have witnessed the effects of pregnancy and child rearing on both women and men, personally and professionally. I have treated three and even four generations of the same family and have an appreciation for the effects of both nature and nurture on who we are as people. With this book and website, my goal is for you to challenge some of the things you take for granted about your body, and to provide a context for how to live physically in a healthy way. Healthcare systems can only succeed if the individuals using them try to help themselves with assertion. This is my way of helping you to help yourself. Enjoy.

# Getting Old Sucks

## Myths to Dispel:

- Age is an excuse

- Genetics are to blame for your problems

- Gravity is your friend

# Human Nature:
# Life as a Journey

On August 19, 2014, I began to truly understand what it meant when people said, "Life is a journey." Up until that point, I thought it was just a phrase like the many others I had heard over my eleven years as a physiotherapist. After my accident, though, it really started to resonate with me, and developed into a meaning that I would like to help others to understand. I always felt that I could empathetically connect with people in pain, because I had managed to hurt most parts of my body over the years, but my appreciation for the impact of life events deepened when I badly injured my right eye that summer.

There is a lot going on under the surface in the human body that most people simply take for granted. The fact that you can effortlessly breathe, see, and move around freely without so much as a thought is part of the miracle of life. Life can be awesome from moment to moment, day to day and even decade to decade, and then all of a sudden become really dark because one aspect that you were taking for granted stops working properly. The life you once knew may get flipped on its head for the foreseeable future, leaving any plans a distant memory. As the notorious Mike Tyson once said, "Everybody has a plan until they get punched in the mouth."

As a physiotherapist, I have worked with people who have been crushed by machines, fallen off roofs, been hit by cars, suffered strokes, and slowly deteriorated with Parkinson's disease, but I don't think I gained a genuine appreciation for the everyday loss that these people dealt with until I lost the functional vision in my eye. I also witnessed my twenty-seven-year-old cousin Sam deteriorate with ALS at the same time. In the span of a year and a half, I underwent seven eye surgeries in attempt to save what was left of my vision; meanwhile, my cousin gradually lost the function of his whole body, piece by piece. I struggled with double vision, headaches, and the loss of the sports I loved, while he lost the ability to breathe and swallow on his own. His battle was obviously more difficult than mine, but his pain didn't ease what I was going through; instead, it made me focus on what I still had going forward.

Communicating with Sam helped me to accept my injury, my loss, and my decreased functionality as a life event that I was just going to have to deal with moving forward. The process of accepting my new state has also helped me to realize just how easy it can be to let pain and injury define who you are, and that falling into a state of depression, resentment and anger can lock you into the past and present, with little hope for the future.

It can be difficult to think beyond the current moment, especially when it takes everything you have just to deal with the pain and discomfort you are facing right then. As a person who professionally deals with people in pain, I have experienced the psychology of trying to create hope and understanding in a person who is lost in the chronic fog of physical dysfunction. Emotion, behavior and fear become entangled with the true source of pain, to the point when you aren't sure which is the bigger problem. Professionally, I have found that people in pain need a sound voice of reason to help them better understand their situation and to instill some logic and hope to help them think forward. Personally, on the other hand, I have found a strong need to avoid harping on my continuing challenges, accept what happened to me, and focus on what I can do to make my tomorrow better than my yesterday.

It is the little things in life that people always focus on when something goes wrong, because these little things are what we take for granted. Most people never consider a life where they can't breathe well, hold themselves up vertically, swallow or see properly, but if you take any of those functions away from somebody, everything changes due to a massive loss of independence, which is replaced with a strong sense of vulnerability. Anybody who has hurt their back and has been stuck on the floor for a period of time can relate to the initial feeling of helplessness, followed by a strange realization of how far away their feet really are when they need to get dressed, followed by the challenge of struggling to brush their teeth. When days of acute pain and dysfunction start turning into weeks and months, it is the acceptance of the continuous reminders of new physical challenges in daily tasks that can help alleviate the depressive thoughts that inevitably dampen the situation.

Only a relative minority of people end up suffering major injuries and illnesses, but the lessons that they are forced to learn and the perspective that they gain on their physical bodies are valuable information to pass on to the general public. Nothing can prepare you for a major accident or illness, but developing an awareness of and connectedness to your body now can help give you the perspective to get through the mental challenges that come with the inevitable deterioration we face with aging.

In my office, I repeatedly see mothers and fathers in their forties and fifties who are trying to be active again after a ten-year lapse due to devotion to their kids. Men want to jump right back into their sports, but after ten years—and ten pounds of muscle being redistributed as twenty pounds of fat around their bodies—they are shocked to discover that they don't move like they once did, and many end up getting hurt. Mothers often fail to fully acknowledge how much the one, two, or three pregnancies changed their bodies, and many think it is normal that they experience incontinence if they go for a jog. Pregnancy and parenthood are major life events on the journey that should not be understated, because they affect everything going forward.

Parents often become parents around age thirty—an age when their invincible years have ended and their bodies are becoming a little higher maintenance. Unfortunately, this new period of their lives, when they should really start paying attention to their own bodies, is completely devoted to looking after the needs of their kids. Being responsible for another human life tends to pull your attention away from your own. The days are long, but the years are short, and pretty soon you are a forty-five-year-old with a bad back, a growing belly, ailing parents, demanding children, and a mortgage to pay. I see people from nine to ninety years old every day, so I work with a broad cross-section of all stages of life, and if there is one group that requires a little heads up of what to expect, it is new parents.

I have gained a great deal of insight on human nature through trying to help people to help themselves. Many of the problems people face with their bodies are, in some way, of their own doing and require a change of behavior on their part. That said, humans are creatures of habit, and change is not always easy. We become hardwired to move and think a certain way, and changes that challenge those ingrained behaviors will face difficulty in sticking unless there is ongoing positive or negative feedback to support them. Physiotherapy exercises are a good example. Most people go to physical therapy expecting some form of treatment and a set of exercises to work on at home, and most people will do their exercises. . . for a while. People will typically do their exercises as long as they are still experiencing pain or dysfunction, and they often stop as soon as they start feeling better. I don't blame them; I would do the same thing. Life is too busy to do things on a regular basis that you don't really want to do.

I started recognizing pretty early in my career as a physiotherapist that there is a large discrepancy in what people think they want for themselves and what they are actually willing to do. I found that teaching clients to perform new exercises was helpful for them, but the usefulness of the new information was short-lived. We were focusing too much on what they should be doing instead of why and how they should be doing it. People are good at following instructions, but in order to empower and motivate them to actually do the work, a strong emphasis must first be placed on helping them understand why. Motivation becomes lost in a sea of uncertainty, but explanations that build a context of why and how people can help themselves usually create the necessary behavior modification.

I found myself giving clients fewer and fewer stretching and strengthening exercises to do at home and spent more time focused on teaching people how to be instead of what to do. Sitting, standing, walking, bending, and breathing differently didn't require more time, they just required more thought. Lack of time was a built-in excuse for people to not do their exercises and provided a justification for their lack of improvement. I decided to get around this unfortunate phenomenon by showing people how life itself should be their workout and how everything else was just a bonus. It doesn't make sense to me how people believe that the five to ten minutes of stretching they perform in a day might have a lasting effect on their bodies, compared to the eight hours they spend poorly sitting or standing at work. I shifted much of my attention to my clients' global posture and movement patterns for day-to-day tasks, and I quickly found they started moving better—even though they might admit they "didn't have time to do their exercises." Connecting what they were learning about their bodies to meaningful tasks in their lives helped clients build better awareness in moving well throughout the day, instead of ignoring their body and then running out of time to do their exercises.

I still give people exercises, but I frame them as motor learning opportunities and demonstrate how they will help specific, everyday tasks. I don't give sets and reps of exercises anymore; instead, I encourage people to practice the posture or movement for one to two minutes and pay attention to how they are doing it, because they need to make the transference to the life task. Once they accomplish this transference of the new skill, it has a way of working into their daily life. At this point I could not care less if they stop doing the exercise. An exercise that only helps you as long as you keep doing it every day for the rest of your life is not a solution to the problem—it is a Band-Aid. Genuine solutions may be harder to earn, but they are much more rewarding accomplishments for both the physiotherapist and the client.

From day one with clients, I preach what I learned in the years working with golfers at Body Balance for Performance: in order to create change in your body, you must go through a process of release, re-educate, rebuild. First, I release tension from their body, typically using intramuscular stimulation (IMS, or dry needling) and/or manual therapy. I then teach them how to move more efficiently so they don't continue to create tension and return to step one. Finally, I help them build strength on top of their new, proper movement patterns instead of their old dysfunction. Many people skip step two and focus on stretching and strengthening with limited and plateauing improvements. The bulk of the work should happen in the second phase to make a long-lasting and preventative change in the body.

Preventative health is a term that is directly linked to human nature and the journey of life. Essentially everyone will agree that it is a good idea, but only few will embrace what it means or how to do it. For example, I am often asked, "How long will the effects of IMS last after treatment?" and my answer is always longer than clients are expecting. The fact that they even asked the question shows a detachment of responsibility for their own body. It may last a couple of hours or a couple of years depending on what was contributing to the pain in the first place. My point is that the person should be asking, "What can I do to make this last?" instead of focusing on when they will need me to fix them again.

I, along with other healthcare professionals, can loosen and straighten you up, but once we release you back into the world with a tuned-up body, it is your job to try and keep it that way for as long as possible. If you find that treatment is really helpful but short-lived, you need to ask yourself what it is you're doing that is creating your pain, both physically and mentally. Stress and anxiety are just as hard on the body as physical labor or sitting at a desk all day, and most people have a combination of factors. The keys to preventative health are knowing yourself, being honest with yourself, and asking for help with the aspects you know you're not strong in.

From my position as an injury-prone, athletic physiotherapist in his mid-thirties with three young children and aging parents, I offer the following groups advice:

**Teenagers:** Be active, play sports, and enjoy your invincible years. Your body is changing quickly, so do your best to learn how to use it properly. If you hurt yourself, use it as an opportunity to discover how your body heals, and see a physiotherapist for advice instead of your family doctor. Pay attention to how your parents and grandparents sit, stand, and move, and pick on them before they pick on you.

**Twenty-somethings:** Your body and your world are becoming your own. Take control of that process mentally, physically, and emotionally. Enjoy your freedom, but set yourself up for success by learning about others and yourself. Your invincibility is weakening, and soon your body will require longer to heal, and it will want more sleep and less alcohol. You are going to need your body for the life you are training for, so take the time to listen to what it is telling you. Occasional trips to the physiotherapist can guide you in the right direction.

**Thirty-somethings:** Marriage and kids are both horribly inconvenient and the best thing ever, wrapped into one package. Prepare yourself for the paradigm shift from your single life so you can dive right in head-first and embrace the awesomeness, because if you don't, you could be stuck resenting the time you should be enjoying. Remember that the best way you can help your kids is to help yourself first. Make a conscious effort to have fun with your spouse and to pay attention to your own body. Life can get in the way of self-care, but you will have to plan ahead, as it is worth it now more than ever. Start paying closer attention to your diet, how much you drink, and consider a monthly visit to a physiotherapist, registered massage therapist, chiropractor, or naturopath to make sure everything is still clicking. Your invincible years are officially over, but life is just beginning!

**Forty-somethings:** Reality usually kicks in by now—if it didn't already in your thirties—that your body doesn't work quite like it used to. You may be sandwiched by teenage kids and ailing parents, not to mention a full-time job. Life stressors can be high at this stage and have an impact on your physical and mental state. Make time to exercise. It will help you feel better, even if you don't think you have the time. Do something you enjoy, not something you hate. Gyms are not for everyone, but there are plenty of other options. Start building a team of allied health professionals around you to keep your body in order and to give you direction going forward. Physiotherapy, massage, counseling, chiropractic, and naturopaths all have their roles in preventative health; your family doctor should be there as back-up. Be assertive in your health.

**Fifty-somethings:** As you will read in the next section, life is a march toward stenosis, and your fifties may be the age when you learn what that word means. Your spine and joints likely have some degenerative change by now and your muscles are getting less elastic. The phrase "use it or lose it" will start to ring true as your body craves a certain amount of movement and exercise. You will need to balance activity with rest days to get the most out of your body, because too little and too much can both have negative effects. A personal trainer or a private Pilates instructor could be a very good investment in your future by helping you reconnect with your body and demonstrating how to exercise safely and regularly. Once a month, tune-ups at the physiotherapist are a good idea.

**Sixty-somethings:** Be assertive in dealing with your mental state and physical health. I notice a substantial discrepancy with people in their sixties and their outlook on life. Some seem to have a foot in the grave while others are thriving, embracing grandparenthood, and either still working or enjoying retirement. Try your best to stay connected with the fast-changing world, and try to consciously mold what you want your next twenty years to look like. Physical mobility is often the key to enjoying your seventies and eighties, so start working on it now if you haven't already. I have taught old dogs new tricks. You may have a body that isn't cooperating with you, but you can always prevent it from getting worse, and likely make it better than you had ever thought possible. Find a group or activity that helps you stay active every week of the year. Your body needs regular maintenance. Work on your balance and leg strengthening at home and with a physiotherapist.

**Seventy and beyond:** At seventy, you are the cumulative product of everything you have done and experienced up to this point. Embrace your wisdom and teach people who are willing to listen. Be stoic in dealing with your health, but be willing to reach out for help. A lot can go wrong with your body and your brain, but not everything is a product of age, and there are people out there who can provide help if asked. Healthcare and technology have improved a lot in your lifetime, so there is no better time to take advantage of it than now. Go for a walk every day.

# Life: A March Toward Stenosis

My favorite part about being a physiotherapist is the perspective I gain by working with a broad array of people: young people, old people, active people, sedentary people, successful people, and those just starting out. I find it fascinating to see the world through these people's eyes as I'm granted glimpses into their lives during our thirty-minute appointments each week. The relationships people have with their own bodies are a very curious thing to me.

Some people literally behave like their bodies are vehicles to walk their head around; they have little-to-no awareness of how or what they are doing physically and are blinded by cognitive factors like stress and anxiety. Others treat their body like a temple and seek help when they detect even the slightest change from their normal, homeostatic state. Many people's relationship with their body is a product of their early childhood experiences combined with their recent fitness endeavors. Your early sports and movement experiences are responsible for molding general postures, while your more recent fitness endeavors have created the lens through which you see your physical self.

Some people choose personal trainers, others choose yoga classes, and some are determined to work out at home with programs like Foundation or P90X. Your choice of physical activity will affect your perception of what physical health means to you. You may become focused on strength, or flexibility, or endurance, or speed. I see many people in my practice who were active as teenagers, but who are now in their early forties with two kids and are trying to rediscover their bodies; unfortunately, many people get hurt during this phase, because their bodies have aged ten to twenty years since last being active, and their choice of activity was based more on familiarity than suitability.

People tend to migrate toward what they are good at when it comes to exercise, but the best results often come from working on improving their areas of weakness. When clients ask me what they should or shouldn't do exercise-wise after I have helped put them back together, my first question is typically, "What would you normally do?" It is important to continue doing what you enjoy, but most people need to find a more efficient, realistic and body-aware way to do it. The main goal of physical exercise should be to challenge your body to move in ways you don't normally in the regular course of the day: reaching up, moving sideways, twisting, bending, lifting something heavy, sweating, breathing deeply, and so on.

The kicker is that the older you get, the more and more attention you need to pay to how you move. As you age, physical health and pain prevention become increasingly about body control and awareness with less emphasis on the quantity of effort. I have encountered numerous sixty-year-olds who had spent the previous ten years doing the same daily stretching routine, but they still couldn't touch their toes. I loosened a couple of things, taught them to move differently and voila—one week later they email me, astounded that they could touch their toes. Awareness plus persistence yields far better results than stubbornness, but unfortunately, that is how most people become as they age—more unwilling to consider changing their postures and physical behaviors.

I teach old dogs new tricks every day. It can be a very rewarding experience for me, and an extremely eye-opening and frustrating, yet positive, experience for my clients. Our bodies are the cumulative product of everything we have put them through, from birth to right now. We start life with the trauma of being pushed, jammed and pulled through the birth canal, then learn how to walk and run in a phase when we have zero regard for our own well-being. We continue to punish our bodies in our invincible teenage years, while we are still structurally developing but are cognitively immature and impressionable. By our mid-twenties to early thirties, our bodies shift from developing to degenerating, and it's at this point when I start hearing the all-so-common phrase in my office: "Getting old sucks."

When I hear "getting old sucks" from a thirty-one-year-old, a forty-five-year-old and an eighty-four-year-old in the same day, it reminds me of how two separate and very experienced healthcare professionals, who have influenced my career, started their seminars. Dr. Chan Gunn and Dr. Shirley Sahrmann both began their multi-day courses with the sentiment that "life is a march toward stenosis." Stenosis is the medical word for the narrowing of the holes in your spine where the nerves pass through, as your spine degenerates over time. It is a significant problem for many seniors from their seventies to their nineties, but an underestimated issue in thirty- to sixty-year-olds.

Your brain and spinal cord are like your fuse box; they are the central control station for the network of nerves that connects every system in your body. It constantly transmits signals to your organs and muscles, as well as back to your brain and spinal cord, to help keep you functioning. Unfortunately, the protective casing of the fuse box must contend with gravity and your attempts to deal with it all day, and after about twenty-five years it begins to slowly break down. The discs in your spine that act as shock absorbers dry up little by little, and your spine's durability as a whole starts to diminish. The joints and ligaments in your spine become overly compressed or stretched due to years of less-than-perfect posture. The car accident you had, combined with the numerous falls or bangs, have created alignment issues and further wear and tear.

Thinning of the discs and small levels of degeneration in the spine will typically not create significant symptoms, but they will combine over time to create increased sensitization of your nervous system, which can affect all of your systems. Your nerves are the electrical wiring to your muscles; if they are annoyed as they pass through your spine, you will be prone to tightness and possibly pain. Your nerves are also the wiring of your organs, so spinal issues can contribute to abdominal problems like an irritable bowel or heartburn. Your organs have vast connections to your brain and spine, which is partly why digestive and emotional issues can grow more prominent as you age.

Long story short, your body starts physically breaking down when you are only about one-third of the way through your life. The speed at which that happens depends largely on how you have treated your spine up to that point and how well you take care of it going forward. There are many important things in life, but they all fade in importance when you can't move around very well. Trust me, I see it every half hour, all day long.

It does suck getting old, as does the reality of your body breaking down year-by-year, but that process is not set in stone by your DNA. Your body will adapt to the forces you place on it, so you are not necessarily destined to suffer the same fate as your parents—if you learn to work with your unique body. Age is not an excuse for pain, but it is a factor. If you want to live a healthy, active lifestyle with minimal pain for decades to come, learn to respect the diminishing tolerances of your body and find your "sweet spot" for the right amount of exercise. Too little exercise may cause stiffness or make you weak; too much may also stiffen you up and cause inflammation. Everyone needs to find their zone in the bell curve of exercise while not extending into their zone of diminishing and damaging returns.

My best advice for thirty- to sixty-five-year-olds wallowing in the discomfort of aging is to strive to develop physical wisdom by means of body awareness and movement experience. Create a connection with your body so you know when it is time to seek help. Pay attention to how you and those around you stand, sit, walk, and move. Compare yourself physically to your parents and your kids, and identify your habitual postures that are less than ideal. If you grow more aware of your body over time, you can start to feel better each year instead of worse.

# Claire's Body: A Vehicle to Walk Her Head Around

In 2006, I met one of the first heads that happened to have a body to walk it around. I was sitting in the treatment room of my new business, Envision Physiotherapy. I had subleased some space from two brothers with a company called Target Personal Training & Health Services; I was the "health services." I had agreed to do free screening consults for their new gym members. It was a means for me to build my caseload while acting as a value-add for the brothers to offer when selling gym memberships to prospective clients.

Claire was one of the first lost souls that I rescued from the grasps of the fitness industry. She was a counselor in her late fifties with two bad hips, daily pain, and a feeling she needed to work out to solve her problems. She twirled into my office, barely escaping the enterprising brother eager to sell her a personal training package at the front desk, and unloaded her story on me. She had already had surgery on both hips—a total hip replacement on one and an osteotomy on the other, but she was still experiencing significant hip and back pain and having trouble with her balance. The doctors insisted that her surgeries were successful, so she was left to her own devices to solve her problems. She decided that joining a gym and getting in shape was her best option, even though she was not a "gym person."

I suggested to her that people who hate the gym should probably not choose going to the gym as their means of change, but we would assess her and go from there. I had her stand up so I could inspect her alignment. She stumbled as she quickly got out of the chair, turned around in the braced, chest up, shoulders back and down, tall posture that she seemed to think I was looking for. I asked her to stand on one leg. She threw her knee up, braced her back, tucked her butt under her and wobbled to stay up, and determination won out; she stayed on one foot. I had her lie down so I could feel her hips. I started to pick up her leg, and it was as if she was trying to guess where I was moving. She braced and tried to help me the whole way, on both sides. Finally, I took her into the gym and asked her to walk to the treadmill and back. She took off like she was being chased. When she returned, I said, "Can you do that one more time a bit slower?" and she said, "Sure," and she proceeded to power across the room in the same manner.

Claire's relationship with her body seemed very black-and-white. It would get her from A to B. Faster was better than slower. More was better than less. She had her way of moving and hadn't considered that there may be other ways; she simply thought that she was in pain because she hadn't done enough. After fifty-eight years of doing it her way, how could I expect her to change? I talked to her about the importance of understanding how her body moves before trying to make it stronger, and that there are shades of gray in how we accomplish something. I helped her to understand that while her determination would facilitate improvements in strength if she trained in the gym, those improvements would plateau and she would likely start hurting herself, because she didn't possess a healthy body awareness. Building strength on top of existing dysfunction only buries the problem even deeper.

As a counselor, Claire was receptive to personal reflection; she just wasn't used to having it focused on her and in a physical way. She agreed in principle with the sentiment of movement being about the journey more than the destination, but she was hardwired to focus on the finish line. I talked her out of joining the gym, much to the brothers' chagrin, and had her come see me every one to two weeks instead. We worked on functional exercises and movement patterns that gave her brain a workout while she moved her body in a new way. Her body awareness improved, but she was still finding the process frustrating. She was also still experiencing some pain, so I referred her to a good clinical Pilates instructor to help reinforce what we had worked on but with a different approach.

One-on-one Pilates was the right place for Claire. She returned to see me about six months later, after spending time in a non-competitive environment with an instructor and equipment designed for learning to appreciate movement and body awareness. Claire had a different air about her. She seemed more in tune with her issues and more confident about her body, even though she was still having trouble. She felt as though she was ready to try my functional exercises again, because Pilates had given her a new perspective on exercise. We worked on breathing, standing, walking, squatting, bending, and lifting. I helped her try to make life itself her workout. Instead of moving through daily routines in such a hurry, I helped her see how there is ample opportunity in a day to live physically. Her previous strategy was to ignore her body all day and then feel guilty about skipping the gym later on, blaming the latter on why her body hurt. Her Pilates instructor and I helped her realize that if she just paid attention to how she performs everyday movements, her need to go to the gym—a place she hated—would simply go away.

As Aristotle said, "We are what we do repeatedly; excellence, then, is not an act, but a habit." Claire learned to live physically by creating new habits and placing more importance on how she was moving rather than what she was doing.

I continued to see Claire over the following eight years for check-ups, treatment, and direction. She ended up having another hip replacement and became an active grandmother, requiring a little help to keep her moving. In her mid-sixties, Claire was much more in control of her physical health than she was in her fifties, all because she understood how her body works. I can proudly say that her head and her body learned to appreciate each other.

# Movement: Your Body is the Car and You are the Driver

Imagine handing the keys of a finely tuned, cherry-red Porsche 911 to a sixteen-year-old boy, a first time driver, and saying, "Have fun!" Now imagine telling him fifteen years later, after he has been in a few accidents, scratched the paint and destroyed the clutch, that he should have driven more carefully, because this is the only car he will ever own for the rest of his life; he will now have to go for regular tune-ups and will probably require an artificial clutch and a titanium tire sometime in the next thirty years. Oh, and your shocks will get worse and worse every year. I hope you had enough fun driving in the first fifteen years to make the next forty years worthwhile! Sorry I didn't teach you to drive better!

We watch our kids struggle to reach the gas pedal for years then blindly let them grind the gears of their own bodies through their adolescence. We put them into sports in key developmental years that, unknowingly, teach them how to move a particular way and which may mold their posture for the rest of their lives. We tell them to stand up straight with little context of what that means, and we start binding their feet with stiff, little shoes before they can even walk. Children are resilient, moldable little sponges that should be given some direction and opportunity to become good drivers in their own bodies. The trouble is that most parents aren't particularly good drivers themselves, and their kids think that they are invincible until they reach their mid-twenties.

While babies can move, little of it is intentional. Most of their movement is created by a series of reflexes that move an entire limb as one unit. The back extensor muscles develop before the abdominals, as the baby must figure out how to lift up its head and arch its back. Once a baby starts to develop some awareness of the world around him, he tries to figure out how to find the manual override for all these reflexes that keep making him smack himself in the face and kick uncontrollably. Anyone who has watched an infant try to pick up a Cheerio and put it in his mouth for the first time will know what I am talking about. Getting his hand to the Cheerio is feat number one, opening his fist is challenge number two, jamming his tightly closed fist all around his face to find his mouth is battle number three and, finally, opening his hand and sticking the Cheerio to the side of his head is the frustrating fourth stage. He starts again and repetition finally brings success!

Movement experience creates movement skill. A variety of movement experiences from a young age create more refined control of one's body. A strict regimen of the same movements may develop talent, but at the same time it can limit the body's potential for a variety of movement skills. The best example is young girls who are put into ballet and gymnastics from the age of three. There is an emphasis on lifting the chest, depressing the shoulders, swaying the back, and toeing out the legs. These are postures that we consider aesthetically nice but are biomechanically awful for your body. These girls are the most likely to tear the ACL in their knee when they play soccer as teenagers. I have been a physiotherapist for thirteen years, and without a doubt the group that experiences the most pain later in life due to their childhood sports are former ballerinas, dancers, and gymnasts.

I believe that one of the reasons men tend to be more athletic than women is largely because their father and brothers wrestled with them as children. It teaches the kid to twist, push, pull, and run—all fundamental movement patterns. Female animals may not be as physically strong as their male counterparts, but they are just as athletic because they receive a similar movement experience in the wild to the males. The best preventative health tool you can give your children is to encourage them to participate in physical play and a variety of sports, and use the times when they injure themselves as opportunities to teach them about their bodies.

Both of my parents were PE teachers when I was young, and both had their fair share of injuries. I always remember my dad saying, "There's nothing more amazing than the human body." Our lives centered around play. I played soccer, baseball, gymnastics, water-skiing, field hockey, swimming, rugby, wakeboarding, volleyball, golf, badminton, and basketball and managed to hurt myself playing every single one of them. I have now treated thousands of clients, including my family, and have had the opportunity to watch my three children learn to sit, walk, and run. The biggest life lesson I have learned and that I am trying to pass on to you is this: don't take your body for granted; learn how to become a better driver, because your shiny new Porsche will eventually feel like a rickety old clunker.

# Bethany the Ballerina: Accountants Don't Pirouette

While I was working in White Rock at Diane Lee & Associates, I met Bethany. She was a thirty-two-year-old accountant and ballet instructor with persistent sciatica that no one seemed to be able to fix for her. She was super-flexible and very strong, but had lived every day with a nagging, aching pain down her right leg to her calf. Before she met me she had tried a chiropractor, a massage therapist, another physiotherapist, and a personal trainer, but nothing seemed to result in a lasting difference. She usually found some relief, but a few hours or a few days later the pain would always resurface.

As good as I may be at "fixing" people's pain, when I hear this type of story I immediately make it very clear to the client that the reason their pain keeps coming back is likely due to something they are doing and not because the treatment didn't last. Some forms of treatment are, without a doubt, more effective than others, but if you have a therapist treat you and largely eliminate your pain for a few days with it always returning, you should probably look inward at your behavior instead of blaming the effects of the treatment as being "only temporary."

Bethany put the pressure on me by saying that I was her last hope, so I explained that there are some things I could do to her to help, some things we would do together, and some things she was going to have to do on her own. She was on board, so I started by loosening up her hips and lower back like many of the professionals had done before me, but then I tried something different. I shifted the focus to what she does all day. Instead of teaching her new tricks and giving her more to do, I analyzed her old tricks and tried to get her doing less. Bethany had been a ballerina since the age of three, and once she passed her prime, she began teaching ballet. Her posture and movement patterns were aesthetically beautiful and graceful, but those are not the qualities you look for in the body of an accountant.

She was an unlikely superhero who crunched numbers by day and bounded across a stage by night. Unfortunately, the aspects that made her an excellent ballerina were detracting from her work as an accountant, because she couldn't sit in her chair all day without leg pain. She was quite loose-jointed, with extremely flexible hamstrings and the "perfect posture" that ballerinas are known for: chest up, shoulders down, toes out. I was, apparently, the first one to challenge Bethany on her posture. I believed the source of her pain was a functional biomechanics issue. Loose-jointed, flexible people are great at moving, but typically have trouble stacking their skeleton up in an efficient way to remain still for prolonged periods of time. Bethany was no exception.

I explained that she needed to be a ballerina when she was doing ballet and a regular civilian the rest of the time. The two entities didn't mix well. Her super-flexible hamstrings, bendy back, and tendency to hold her trunk up with her shoulders were actually making it harder for her to sit all day. Her perfect posture wasn't so perfect after all. Using a skeleton and anatomy charts, I showed her that the way she was holding herself all day was creating mechanical strain on her lower back, hips, and sciatic nerve. Her subconscious daily postures were also creating tension, irritation, and pain in her body. She sought help to relieve the pain when it grew unmanageable, but she never properly addressed the root issue: how she was standing and sitting all day would restart the cycle of pain each time she left the therapist's office.

Instead of sending her home with exercises, I assigned her with the task of paying attention to how she held her mid back throughout the day. I asked her to start looking at her side profile in the mirror and to start watching how everyone else holds themselves up in different situations. Everyone has their own strategy and Bethany's needed some refining. Her homework was to create some awareness that how she had been moving since she was a child may need to change a little if she wanted her pain to go away. Being a dancer familiar with the nuances of subtle movement corrections, she accepted my challenge.

Bethany came in once a week for about three months, and I slowly trained her how to control the dancer in her. I taught her about what it means to be hypermobile. I showed her how to use her muscles to stack her spine in a stronger position for sitting and standing. I explained why her hamstrings were actually too flexible and that she should stop stretching them, even though they felt tight. I simply helped her change the paradigm of where she felt her body should be in space while performing a variety of tasks like standing, sitting, walking, and bending. What I showed her went against everything her ballet teachers and her mother had preached to her from a young age, but her reinforcement came in the form of decreasing pain each week. I taught her how to make the treatments last.

Many of the principles that I taught Bethany may be relevant to you. Some people are hypermobile, some aren't. Some people stand funny, others sit strangely. There are different ways to breathe, walk, and run. You should find more meaningful explanations in the pages to come and in the videos on WhyThingsHurt.com.

# Being Hypermobile: A Gift and a Curse Wrapped in One

I grew up as a long and lanky kid playing every sport that was available to me. I loved team sports, especially soccer and rugby. If I knew then what I know now about my body, I would have stuck to volleyball and swimming. Don't get me wrong, I thoroughly enjoyed the sports I played, but I routinely felt like I had been hit by a truck after every game, and I still have two wonky shoulders to prove it.

I am what you would call hypermobile: this means that the soft tissues that help hold my skeleton and joints together are relatively looser and more flexible than the average person's. It is a genetic trait that a large number of people have, but most have no concept that the way they are put together is not "normal." It does go both ways, as some people are deemed hypomobile, implying that their spine and joints are relatively stiffer than the average population. Everyone falls somewhere on the spectrum of joint mobility based on the genetically determined amount of proteins in your soft tissues, called elastin. Some hit the genetic lottery of having just the right balance, while others fall into the Goldilocks trap of too much or too little.

The chart below is my estimation of the incidence of pain and injury as they correlate to genetic joint mobility:

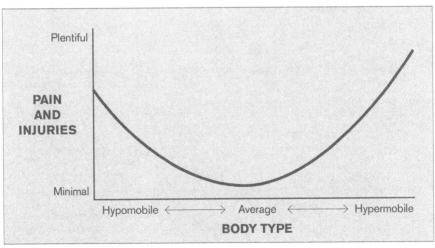

This chart shows the relation of pain and injuries to the different body types.

Being loose-jointed may sound like a positive genetic attribute, but let me assure you that it can pose plenty of problems. Gravity can become particularly annoying when you are hypermobile, especially if you have a job that requires you to sit or stand still for any length of time. We are the only creatures on Earth that are built to stand and walk upright on two feet; this biomechanical feat requires a skeleton that provides both structural stability to vertically stack your body and functional mobility so that you can move freely. Hypermobile people are built to move and have to work much harder than everyone else to stack everything up and stay still. We are also the only creatures on Earth that attempt to sit at desks or stand at counters for eight hours at a time.

When the passive support structures that hold you together are relatively loose, you become a lot more reliant on your muscular system, which can be both a good and a bad thing. A hypermobile body is physically capable of many more movements and positions than its hypomobile counterpart, but it will fall into the paradox of choice: if your body has twenty different postures to choose from, finding the right one can be difficult. Control of your muscular system requires learned skill in order to use it and move it well, and most hypermobile people never develop enough awareness to control their loosey-goosey bodies. As a result, they tend to develop strong muscle imbalances and postural issues, and are susceptible to some very common aches and pains if they attempt to function at a desk job or do physical labor.

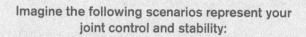

### Imagine the following scenarios represent your joint control and stability:

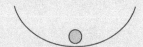

| Scenario 1: Normal/Average Person | Scenario 2: Hypomobile/Stiff Person | Scenario 3: Hypermobile/Loosey-Goosey Person |
|---|---|---|
| *Task:* I give you a marble and a small bowl and ask you to move the marble around the bowl, then try to balance it right in the middle. | *Task:* I give you the same marble but instead a shot glass and ask you to move the marble around then try to balance it right in the middle. | *Task:* I give you the same marble and this time a huge mixing bowl and ask you to move the marble around then try to balance it right in the middle. |
| *Result:* You will have some room to play with it and not much trouble keeping it in the middle. | *Result:* You won't have much movement, but it's much easier to keep it centered. | *Result:* You will have plenty of fun moving the marble all around the bowl, but you are going to have trouble finding the middle because you have so much room to move. |

 The marble analogy is used to compare how joint control and stability works in the three different body types.

Consider the marble analogy scenario happening at every level of your spine, in your hips, your knees, and throughout your body. Stiff people are good at standing still, carrying heavy loads, and pushing big objects because their bodies provide them with a genetic mechanical advantage, while loose-jointed people are good movers but find the seemingly simple task of sitting still very difficult. Some people are built to be accountants while others are meant to be ballerinas. We run into trouble when the ballerina wants to become an accountant, or the accountant wants to become a ballerina. Then there was me—the six-foot-five, loose-jointed rugby player whose shoulder fell out every time he tackled someone. I became a physiotherapist to figure out how to put my body back together and keep it that way.

Clinically speaking, treating the most hypermobile of people can be challenging, because it is like trying to solve a three-dimensional moving puzzle; each time you see them they may move differently than the time before, and you are forced to chase the problem around while teaching them how to create some control and awareness in their bodies. As I mentioned, hypermobile people are much more dependent on their muscular system for stability: this makes them more vulnerable to having muscle imbalances, which creates problems with their alignment. If they have a fall on one hip or are whiplashed in a car accident, the resulting muscle spasm will likely cause them more trouble than your average person. It can also be much harder to detect imbalances, because the person may still have a wide range of movement compared to the average person, but slight differences in muscle pulls can throw their stability system out of whack.

Stiff, hypomobile people generally gain a substantial benefit simply by loosening them up and decompressing everything, but hypermobile people must put in a great deal more cognitive effort and practice to learn the skills of using their muscular system correctly. It is the hypermobile people with poor body awareness who tend to have chronic pain issues most often and have the hardest time recovering from even minor car accidents.

Understanding your body type is a crucial step to proper rehabilitation of an injury and the prevention of future pain. Just because you may feel stiff all the time does not mean you are hypomobile; in fact, hypermobile people tend to experience the most stiffness out of any group. I recommend seeing a healthcare practitioner who is used to working with people's bodies, such as a physiotherapist, Pilates instructor, massage therapist, or chiropractor, and ask for some feedback about your joints, muscles, and fascia (connective tissue).

# Why Hips Hurt:
# An Illustrated Explanation

Why does your hip hurt if you didn't do anything to injure it?

The short answer: You probably harmed it in a whole slate of ways, every day for years, and had no idea that you were doing something wrong.

The full answer: Read below.

Your hips are the center of your universe. They are the connection of your upper and lower body, and most people have no idea where they are or how to use them properly. It is strange to suggest that someone doesn't know where his own hips are, but take it from a guy who teaches people to move all day: most people have trouble distinguishing their hips from their pelvis or how to move in a strong, coordinated way through their midsection.

There are more moving parts in your body than you have the capacity to focus on at any given time, so the best way to explain this is to simplify your body down to two pieces, adding on layers as you understand. Begin by thinking of your body as two wooden blocks with a round hinge connecting them in the middle. Now remember that gravity pulls everything downward, so imagine trying to balance the upper piece on the round hinge by holding onto the lower piece. There are three likely scenarios:

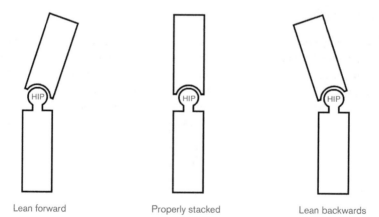

Lean forward          Properly stacked          Lean backwards

To bring these pictures to life, let's add a head and neck and see what happens. You must also understand that your brain has a head-righting reflex that wants to keep your head and face looking straight forward, so if one part of your body is persistently leaning one direction your head and neck will accommodate for it.

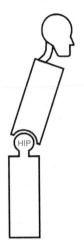 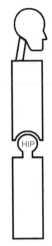 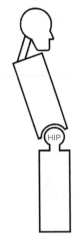

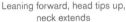

| Leaning forward, head tips up, neck extends | Properly stacked, neck supported over body | Leaning backward, head and neck jutting forward |

So far we have block men with hips and necks, an upper body, a lower body, and a head. The above illustrations are three common postural types, but we all know the human body has more joints in it. Let's first add an upper body hinge. Your spine has twenty-four vertebrae, all with their own hinges, but the most common hinging point is around the middle of your torso. So let's add one hinge there and see what happens to the posture.

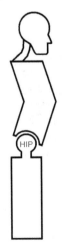 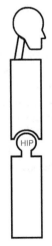 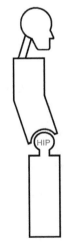

| Upper torso leans back, lower torso tips forward, head remains relatively over top of hips | Body remains in neutral stacked position | Upper torso remains straight, lower torso tips backward, head remains over hips |

In these illustrations, you can see where people would be prone to becoming very tight in certain areas based on their posture. The further a person tends to deviate from the straight, "good" posture, the harder time they will have in moving properly with their big hip hinges and the more they will beat up on their joints over time.

Let's now give our block people knees and see what happens:

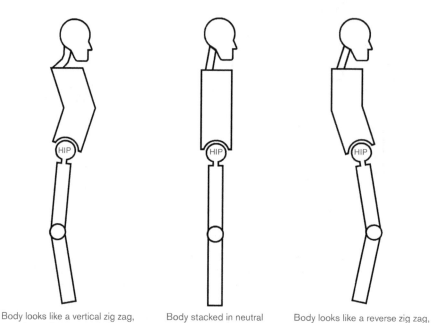

| Body looks like a vertical zig zag, knees hyperextended | Body stacked in neutral alignment, efficiently dealing with gravity | Body looks like a reverse zig zag, knees held flexed |

The people who aren't properly stacked will be very prone to developing chronic tension in specific areas due to overuse from dealing with gravity and trying to stay vertical. It is hard to coordinate all the moving parts properly so people will tend to overly brace a certain area in their body as their strategy to hold themselves up. Some people hold all their tension in their butt, others their back, some their stomach or chest. It is helpful to identify where a person "grips" most and make them aware of their bracing strategy so they can work on toning it down. Improving posture requires first addressing the bad habits before introducing new ones.

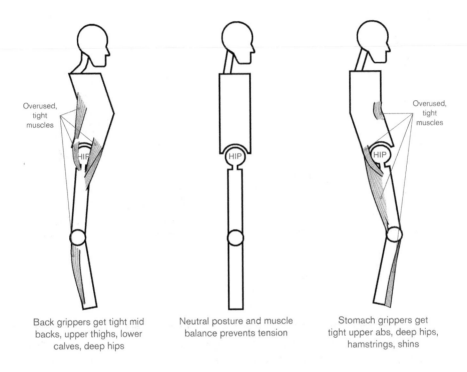

Back grippers get tight mid backs, upper thighs, lower calves, deep hips

Neutral posture and muscle balance prevents tension

Stomach grippers get tight upper abs, deep hips, hamstrings, shins

You may be able to tell from the illustrations above that how you tend to hold your upper body will impact how you hold your lower body, and vice-versa; the hips are stuck in the middle with the purpose of keeping you vertical. More often than not, the root cause of hip issues is a product of body posture as a whole.

That being said, let's give our people a pelvis, ankles and feet. The pelvis can tip anteriorly or posteriorly to add a layer of complexity to your center, while your entire posture can be thrown off by shoes with various heights of a heel.

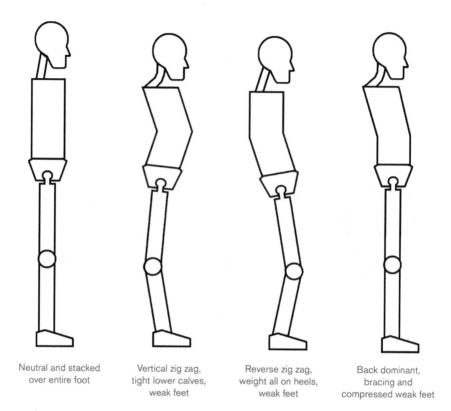

Neutral and stacked
over entire foot

Vertical zig zag,
tight lower calves,
weak feet

Reverse zig zag,
weight all on heels,
weak feet

Back dominant,
bracing and
compressed weak feet

By now you are likely getting the picture of how posture can affect your hips, but let's take a closer look at how these postures actually create pain. The hip is happiest when functioning deep in the middle of the socket. Ideally your pelvis balances on top of both hips in a slightly tipped-forward position, and the muscles on every side of the hip work in a coordinated tug-of-war to keep everything balanced. Unfortunately, as we will see in the illustrations on the next page, the upper and lower body don't always come together in a balanced way, and the hip joint is levered one way or the other.

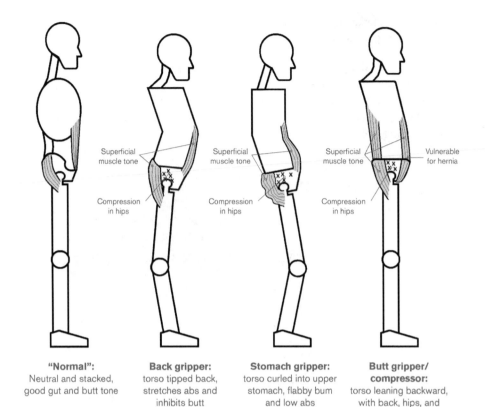

| Superficial muscle tone | | Superficial muscle tone | | Superficial muscle tone | | Vulnerable for hernia |
| Compression in hips | | Compression in hips | | Compression in hips | | |

| **"Normal":** | **Back gripper:** | **Stomach gripper:** | **Butt gripper/ compressor:** |
|---|---|---|---|
| Neutral and stacked, good gut and butt tone | torso tipped back, stretches abs and inhibits butt | torso curled into upper stomach, flabby bum and low abs | torso leaning backward, with back, hips, and upper abs braced |

In "good" or "normal" posture, your butt (gluteus maximus) works together with your abdominals, and your back works together with your thighs. Your gluteus maximus (the bigger part of your butt) functions optimally when your body is nicely erect. If your pelvis is too tipped forward or too tipped backward due to postural issues, the gluteus maximus won't work properly. The result is overactivity of the deep muscles underneath, namely your gluteus medius, piriformis and adductors (inner thigh); these smaller muscles have to work harder to hold the ball in the socket when the glutes aren't firing properly, and typically the result is significant trigger points and muscular pain. The joint can get over-compressed in the socket and/or tend to pinch and rub in the front of the joint. Over time, this pattern of muscle-overactivity and poor movement can lead to wear and tear in the joint, sciatica, pelvic dysfunctions, lower-back pain, torn labrums, and, eventually, advanced osteoarthritis.

In order to have good posture and normal-functioning hips, the various parts of your body must work together in a coordinated, strong manner that provides stability and mobility throughout your joints. Unfortunately, due to learned behavior as a child, genetics, sports, pregnancy, accidents, work, and personality, we develop a variety of muscle imbalances and postural strategies that may predispose us to pain and injury over time. The tendency is for people to latch on to one or two areas of their body to hold everything up at the expense of everything else.

My colleague Diane Lee first introduced me to the concept of "butt grippers," "back grippers," and "stomach grippers." Look at the pictures in this section, and then stand and look at your side profile in a full-length mirror, choosing which one most resembles you. These pictures are not all-encompassing, but they demonstrate the majority of people's body types.

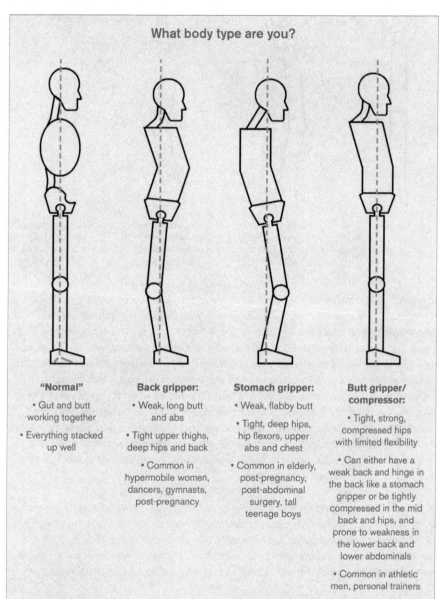

## What body type are you?

**"Normal"**
- Gut and butt working together
- Everything stacked up well

**Back gripper:**
- Weak, long butt and abs
- Tight upper thighs, deep hips and back
- Common in hypermobile women, dancers, gymnasts, post-pregnancy

**Stomach gripper:**
- Weak, flabby butt
- Tight, deep hips, hip flexors, upper abs and chest
- Common in elderly, post-pregnancy, post-abdominal surgery, tall teenage boys

**Butt gripper/ compressor:**
- Tight, strong, compressed hips with limited flexibility
- Can either have a weak back and hinge in the back like a stomach gripper or be tightly compressed in the mid back and hips, and prone to weakness in the lower back and lower abdominals
- Common in athletic men, personal trainers

These are the most common postures, but people tend to mix-and-match to find creatively bad ways to hold themselves up. I always like to remind people that just because they can stand, sit, walk, and run does NOT mean that they do these things very well. Your body is fantastic at cheating and compensating during movement, and the more it cheats, the more your body parts will start to break down and hurt over time; this is very much the case with your hips.

Start paying attention to how other people around you stand; try to recognize the butt grippers and back grippers. Look for long big bums and flat saggy bums. Watch how many people tend to actually lean backward as they stand or walk. It may be difficult to change how you move, but watching others around you will give you a keen eye to learn about yourself. No matter what your posture is or how much pain you may have, there is likely a way to significantly improve it. The best way to start is by following these steps:

1. Start watching other people and practice identifying different body types. Then watch my videos "How to Stand" and "How to Sit" on WhyThingsHurt.com.

2. Look at the drawings in this article and pick which one you think best captures your posture.

3. Determine if you are hypermobile, average, or hypomobile.

4. Watch my video titled "Everything Your Mother Taught you about Posture is WRONG" on WhyThingsHurt.com.

5. Start learning how to move by discovering your hips. There are video exercise progressions on WhyThingsHurt.com.

6. Consider finding a physiotherapist who offers intramuscular stimulation (IMS) to help release tension in your tight areas. This will help with pain and posture, making the entire process easier and faster.

I continue to prove on a daily basis that forty- to sixty-year-olds with chronic posture and pain problems can and should be helped. It is never too late to improve your posture or, at the very least, prevent it from getting even worse. The first step is understanding that what you believe to be "normal" may not be the best way to function, and to start creating awareness of your own body. Your hips are the center of your universe, and although you can technically have them replaced, you will only continue the damaging cycle if you don't address the root cause of how you wrecked the original pair. Take care of your hips by minding your posture and you will have fewer physical issues throughout life.

# Your Invincible Years are Over: How to Stay Strong, Fit, and Pain-free as You Age

I used to beat the hell out of my body when I was in high school. I played soccer, basketball, rugby, and a variety of other sports on an almost-daily basis. I would bang and crash and hurt myself, but it never really slowed me down because I just took it for granted that within a few days or a few weeks my body would heal up and be ready for more. In university, I tested my body with little sleep, even more sports, and a lot of alcohol but I still bounced back and kept going. Then a few things happened that started changing my perspective on life.

By the age of twenty-four, I had completed two university degrees and was officially a registered physiotherapist. I'd like to think I was more intelligent after six years of university, but I learned much more in the following six to ten years than I ever did in school. It was a time when my body was becoming less and less invincible, and I gained more and more perspective on the importance of my physical health. I still played soccer, hockey and squash, but my body was taking longer and longer to recover; problems that used to take days to recover starting taking weeks, and I was forced to consider the physical consequences of my activity choices more than ever.

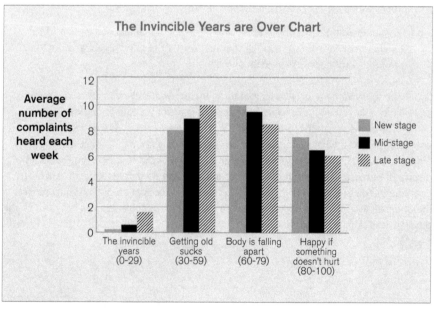

 This chart represents the type and number of complaints heard from my clients during an average week, according to age group.

As a physiotherapist working with clients of all ages, I started recognizing that I was not alone in the weakening of my invincibility around age thirty. I would hear an average of ten "getting old sucks" complaints a week, equally spread among the thirty-, forty- and fifty-year-olds. The sixty- and seventy-year-olds tended to phrase it more around "this old body is falling apart," and the eighty- to ninety-year-olds seemed happy enough if something actually didn't hurt. Thirty seems to be the age when people's cognitive self-awareness improves, responsibilities grow, and financial and emotional stressors hit new highs—all while their bodies are beginning to decline. It is a perfect recipe for injuries and pain.

The following is the typical mindset I try to create in my clients to help take them from a place of pain and stiffness to a place of comfort, control, awareness, and health in their bodies:

**Principles to understand:**

1. Understand what genetics has given you to work with (nature).

2. Appreciate what you have done with what genetics has given you (nurture).

3. Analyze other people's postures and movements and reflect on your own.

4. Think about what you enjoy doing physically and make time for it, then stop feeling bad for not doing things that you hate (like going to the gym).

5. Learn how to live physically by paying attention to how you stand, sit, walk, bend, lift, and move.

6. Understand that your body and your brain require maintenance; develop a network of people around you for support.

7. Nutrition is important: what you put in your body will affect how you feel.

**Understand what genetics has given you to work with (nature)**

Some people win the genetics lottery and others, unfortunately, get the short end of the stick. Some people are naturally gorgeous while others "have a good personality." Some people naturally have an incredible metabolism and can eat whatever they want while others manage to gain weight eating salad and dry toast. Life is not fair, but you can make the most of what you have—if you actually understand what you have.

Life has a blunt way of letting you know if you happen to be stereotypically "hot or not", overweight or slight, but it can be difficult to understand how your body is genetically held together. As we grow up, we assume that we are all built the same, but this is only partially true. For the most part, we all have the same pieces, but how they are all held together can vary significantly from person to person. There are about 360 joints in your body. Imagine how your life would change if I immediately made all of them significantly looser. To stand up and move, your body must coordinate all those joints; do you think it would be easier or harder to move with loose joints? Now imagine I immediately made all of your joints twice as stiff; some activities would be easier and some would be a lot harder.

Everyone and their genetics fall somewhere on the spectrum of hyper or hypomobility. It is related to the amount of a protein called elastin that is present in your tissues; due to genetics, some people's soft tissues become very stretchy and others less so. As you can imagine, there are pros and cons to being on either end of the spectrum, but most people are best suited to fall right in the middle. Unfortunately, as is the case with genetics, you don't get a choice, so you need to learn how to make the most of what you have been given to make healthy decisions about the sports, activities, and careers you choose.

**Appreciate what you have done with what genetics has given you (nurture)**

In the same way a good personality won't get you very far in your modeling career, being hypermobile doesn't do wonders for your dreams of being a pro football player— or a desk jockey, for that matter. Hypermobile people excel in sports and jobs that allow them to move freely, but they soon fall apart when asked to sit at a desk, carry heavy objects all day, or tackle moving targets. Conversely, hypomobile people are good at staying still but shouldn't set their sights on running a marathon.

The trouble is, we want to do what we want to do, regardless of what hand genetics has dealt us. This is actually what keeps me busy as a physiotherapist. I regularly see loosey-goosey accountants, receptionists and lawyers who are having trouble sitting at their desk all day, as well as a surprising number of shapes and sizes deciding to take on the Ironman triathlon as their new challenge. I am tasked with trying to fix the damage they may have done, followed by helping them use their unique body more efficiently to do what they want to do, even though they might not be built for it.

Only on a few occasions have I bluntly told a client that they should pick another sport or career, because their body just wouldn't tolerate the punishment they were doling it. On a daily basis, however, I challenge my clients to stop taking their bodies for granted and remind them that they are the product of everything they have experienced from birth to the present day. Genetics provides you with the platform to work with, but your body reacts to the forces and stresses you put on it. Your current pain, posture, and flexibility are reflections of your past, and how you choose to sit, stand, walk, breathe, and move today will determine how you feel in the future.

**Analyze other people's postures and movements and reflect on your own**

It is difficult when someone challenges how you carry out an activity that you have taken for granted for as long as you can remember. The first time I start analyzing a person's posture, I try to encourage her to see in a mirror what I am talking about. I don't ask her to go out and try to change everything about how she holds herself; instead, I ask her to be aware of what I pointed out and to start analyzing the posture of other people around her.

Most people simply stand how they stand and walk how they walk without much thought, so it becomes cumbersome to change something for which they don't have a strong awareness. Start watching how people stand in line-ups, bus stops, and coffee shops. Look how people walk in flip-flops, running shoes, or high heels. You will notice that some look and move like you and some look much different, yet they are all able to function in this world—some better than others.

You will also begin to notice that some people stand with their feet crossed, some stand with their pelvis in front of them, some people's butt sticks way out behind them, and others have their head way in front of their body. These postures have evolved from how each person, as a child, developed a strategy to vertically hold together all of his or her 360 joints, as well as how they have been molded by watching their parents, their anxieties and stresses at school, the muscular demands of their chosen sports, and the injuries that they have suffered along the way.

You may have been a hypermobile girl who started dance classes at age three and developed a big sway-back, then were embarrassed when you developed breasts earlier than your friends in school and slouched your shoulders and trunk forward to hide them, becoming later in life a lawyer who likes to run. All of those experiences have molded how you subconsciously move today, for better or worse. If you are experiencing pain and stiffness that you just can't seem to resolve, or if physiotherapy, chiropractic treatment, or massage only ever seem to yield temporary relief, you most likely need to reflect on what you are doing with your body all day, because you are what you do repeatedly. It's never too late to change things in your body—it just takes awareness, persistence, and a little help.

**Learn how to live physically by paying attention to how you stand, sit, walk, bend, lift and move**

Remaining vertical all day is itself a form of exercise, because gravity is constantly trying to flatten you into the ground. There is a reason that all of the other animals on Earth don't walk erect like we do: because it's difficult! There are mechanical advantages to being vertical, but it also makes us more susceptible to the unrelenting forces of gravity. I often tell people that "sitting at your desk all day can be harder on your body than a contact sport," and I believe it to be true if the person has no awareness of how he is holding himself for eight-plus hours a day.

Some people are overly sedentary and would likely gain the most benefit from encouragement to increase their movement. Most people, however, move a reasonable amount and would be most helped by learning to move more efficiently. Others, meanwhile, actually move too much and could take a lesson from African lions on lying around and doing nothing once in a while—sometimes less is more. I like to focus on the larger middle group that thinks that they need to do more but stresses that they don't have time, when all they really need to do is start living physically.

There is ample opportunity to turn your day-to-day activities into a form of exercise. Rising and sitting in chairs, bending down to pick things up, sitting on the toilet, lifting your kids, climbing stairs, carrying your groceries—the list goes on. The trouble is, your body is inherently lazy and will always cheat to take the path of least resistance in how you move. Your subconscious brain will allow you to move in a coordinated way, but your conscious brain will do a way better job if you learn how to use it.

Discovering how to find and use the manual override function of your movement autopilot will help you to live physically. Moving properly will likely be more challenging for some time, both physically and cognitively, because you will be fighting against your old movement patterns and muscle imbalances. If you persist through the initial frustration, however, you will find that you become more flexible and stronger, and your body will hurt less without you having to do more. Learn how to use your legs and core to squat and bend. Learn how to breathe well. Learn how to hold yourself up by using your skeleton more than your muscles and ligaments. Discover what your feet can do. Reach up more. Think, and be aware.

Once you have a solid understanding of how to use your body during your day-to-day life, you will be ready to push it further with strength and endurance training. The best way to get hurt while exercising is to ignore your body all day and then try to make it stronger or faster for one to two hours of exercise. In my experience, the fourteen hours of awareness in daily tasks outweighs the benefit of one hour of fitness. In fact, the single hour of fitness without the body awareness is commonly detrimental by further enforcing poor movement patterns and muscle imbalances. You will have a better long-term outcome by addressing your daily movements and postures before pursuing fitness.

**Think about what you enjoy doing physically and make time for it, then stop feeling bad for not doing things that you hate (like going to the gym)**

Lack of flexibility is not directly proportional to how much you stretch, just as a lack of "fitness" is not proportional to how much you go to the gym. If you hate going to the gym, don't go to the gym, but do find something physical that you enjoy doing. If you hate stretching, learn to move well and you probably won't need to stretch.

Health and well-being are lifestyles. We tend to make time for the things in life we enjoy, and we tend to make excuses for the things we don't. If you want to be successful at improving your health, start by paying attention to how you perform your everyday activities. Look in a mirror more, think about how you sit down and rise from your chair, take the stairs, and start keeping notes about what you are doing and turn those notes into goals for habits to change. There is ample opportunity in a day to live physically, but most people will unknowingly migrate to the lazy option.

Most people will feel better physically and emotionally after physical exercise, so find the one you like and go with it, regardless of what others are doing.

**Understand that your body and your brain require maintenance; develop a network of people around you for support**

Preventative health is all about awareness and maintenance. Consider your body a machine that needs occasional tune-ups, both physically and cognitively, and recognize that you can't do that entirely yourself. You have to do most of it on your own, but you will likely need some guidance and treatment to keep you going in the right direction; your doctor should only be a part of this team, not the leader. A couple of allied health practitioners like a good physiotherapist, a massage therapist, and maybe a personal trainer should be able to handle the physical aspects, while a naturopath or nutritionist would be beneficial in addressing your physiologic needs.

On the cognitive side, I believe the type of professional you need depends greatly on your past. People with a fair amount of emotional baggage related to their family life can benefit from semi-regular visits with a counselor to help them understand how their past is affecting their bodies, both at present and in the future. Cognitive issues like stress and anxiety wreak havoc on your body, but both can be addressed when a person is ready and willing to deal with them. I also believe people need a friend, relative, or professional associate to play a mentor role in their lives to help provide direction and to assist in setting goals for the future. I see too many people in pain who are mentally caught in the present or past and just need someone to help them look forward, breaking the cycle of pain and, in many cases, the accompanying depression.

That may sound as if a lot of professionals are required, but you don't have to utilize them all at once. Build relationships with allied health workers so you can call on them when needed, and if something goes wrong you will feel supported in knowing you will get through it. Don't rely on doctors to fulfill all of these roles, because they simply cannot and you will just resent them in misunderstanding their role. Speaking from experience with my clients, the people who have built a network around them tend to live happier and healthier lives, with less stress and pain to interfere.

**Nutrition is important: what you put in your body will affect how you feel**

I will be the first to admit that nutrition is not my area of expertise; that being said, I have a growing awareness of how important a role food sensitivity can play in people's pain, energy, and overall well-being. The further I delve into the world of visceral manipulation (physically treating your organs), the more I consider different foods as irritants to the body. I have come to understand the connectivity of your digestive tract to your nervous system, and now—more than ever—I question my clients about their diet.

Consider talking to a holistic nutritionist, naturopath, or simply start reading on the subject.

**In closing**

In the end, it is your body and you get to choose what you do with it, but trust me when I say that it is never too late to make improvements. Age is just a number, and I have seen countless clients completely change their posture, improve their movement, and manage their pain well into their retirement years.

This book and my website are set up to help you learn something about yourself by reading and watching videos, but I hope it also inspires you to reflect on your relationship with your body and to start implementing some small changes.

# Take Aways and Resources

## Take Aways

→ Life is a journey, so you should treat it like one. Take a step back and look at yourself and your path as objectively as you can in order to not take yourself or your situation too seriously.

→ Acknowledge the reality that your body slowly degenerates over time, and be prepared to make adjustments for it, both physically and mentally.

→ Create awareness in your body from time to time by paying attention to how you do things.

→ Understand that although we all generally have the same parts, we can be held together somewhat differently. You may be genetically hypermobile, and if so it is beneficial to pay closer attention to your posture.

## Websites

✦ WhyThingsHurt.com: written articles with embedded educational and exercise videos, as well as a video library with playlists specific to different body parts.

✦ YouTube.com/user/envisionphysio: my channel of "learning" and "doing" videos that are also embedded on my site.

✦ EnvisionPhysio.com: my Vancouver-based multidisciplinary clinics.

# Understanding Healthcare

## Myths to Dispel:

- Your doctor understands pain

- X-rays, MRIs, and CT scans are always helpful

- It is the medical system's role to fix you

# Pain and Function: What Doctors Don't Understand, and What Patients Don't Understand About Doctors

I have immense respect for doctors and their knowledge base. They go through rigorous training in medical school to learn how the body works, how to fix it when it is broken, and how to keep it alive when it is dying. On a daily basis, doctors help their patients with a wide variety of medical issues, from diabetes to cancer and pregnancy to Parkinson's. We need them in our lives because our society just cannot function properly without them. That being said, I would like to share my personal experience in dealing with doctors from the perspective of an experienced physiotherapist.

The purpose of this article is not to make doctors look bad; it is to help the general public understand what they should and should not expect from their family doctors and the medical system as a whole. Like all medical professionals, doctors are intelligent people, but they don't know everything; most of the time they work in a model that does not allow them to help you in a thorough or timely manner. We should not grow frustrated at doctors for this; instead, we should adjust our expectations and understand that a doctor may not always be the best option to treat our ailments.

When something hurts for a couple of days or weeks without relief, most people search the Internet for their symptoms, and often visit their doctor to figure out what is going on; the focus tends to remain on what is the problem. The patient feels temporarily satisfied because their doctor has given them a name or "diagnosis" for their pain and prescribed a drug for the symptoms, but this satisfaction with what wears off when the patient realizes that it still hurts and they don't understand why. As a physiotherapist, clients routinely hand me their doctor's diagnosis written in chicken scratch on one of their referral pads. Many clients feel as if that little piece of paper is gospel, and now that their doctor has "solved the problem" and found a diagnosis, my job will be that much easier in trying to fix them.

In reality, most family physicians' knowledge level about musculoskeletal pain and injury is based on a combination of their personal experience and limited training in medical school. I have found that most General Practitioners (GPs) will simply diagnose their patients' aches and pains with the most common issue that affects an area, like tendonitis, bursitis, or epicondylitis; "itis" just means inflammation of a particular tissue, so they have effectively used a fancy word to tell you that your body part is swollen.

Mechanical lower-back pain is another common diagnosis that just implies your back hurts when you move. Patellofemoral syndrome is a diagnosis that makes pain around the kneecap sound like a menacing illness for no particular reason. My favorite ailment, though, is when people tell me that they have been diagnosed with TMJ; TMJ stands for temporomandibular joint. It is a joint in your body called your jaw, and not a diagnosis of any meaning. I have to shake my head when I picture a patient going into their doctor's office with jaw pain and coming out with TMJ disorder. Does changing the name of the body part from a layman's term to a medical term and stamping the word "syndrome" or "disorder" on the end help anything? People with chronic pain conditions fall into the medical trap of jargon too. Telling a person what they have without an explanation of why can provide an external label on which to blame their pain, resulting in even worse outcomes. If you are in pain, you need a meaningful explanation to get you engaged in the solution, instead of only labeling the problem.

These diagnoses should, and usually will, come with a referral to a physiotherapist, massage therapist, or chiropractor, because they are deemed "soft tissue" injuries and fall outside of the doctor's area of expertise. As a rule, you should not assume that your doctor knows a great deal about your injury beyond what to call it. They may know more than you about anatomy, injury and healing, but that does not necessarily mean they know why you developed pain or how you should treat it. They do know that rest and painkillers will likely make you feel better, but you are much better to enlist the help of an expert whose training has been specifically focused on pain, injury and rehabilitation, such as a physiotherapist. Most family physicians will readily admit that a physiotherapist's knowledge base is far superior to their own regarding orthopedic pain issues—that is why they refer people to them.

In most places around the world, physiotherapy is considered primary care, which means you do not need a doctor's referral. In Canada, a visit to the doctor's office is covered by your government healthcare plan, but a visit to the physiotherapist's office may cost you some money, so the tendency is visit the doctor first. This process costs our healthcare system a great deal of money, and patients a great deal of their time. Starting with the healthcare professional who likely knows the most about your condition will save you time and your government money. Your physiotherapist will advise you if medical attention is necessary, but in most cases it is best to remain outside of the standard medical system.

Your doctor learns, down to the cellular level, how every system in your body works, but never learns how the body as a whole should actually move. They can probably explain more to you about the physiology of how a muscle contracts than how your shoulder actually functions. They can likely explain how Tylenol relieves pain, but it's doubtful that they could teach you the proper way to stand, sit, walk, or run. We are active, dynamic beings who ask a lot of our bodies on a daily basis. We sit at desks or stand at counters all day. We lift, bend, push, pull, and walk just to get through daily life, but medicine tends to treat us like a collection of static pieces. Doctors know how to assess the pieces when broken, using X-rays and MRIs, and they know how to put them back together in surgery, but they don't really understand how we use all the pieces together to function or how one piece genuinely affects another; that is what physiotherapists understand.

Doctors strongly support the notion of "evidence-based practice" or the idea that their actions are guided by sound research. Most people would agree with this premise, but the major drawback for me is that it creates a bias toward the practices that are easier to research and produce high levels of evidence, medications, and surgeries in particular. I find it tends to make doctors very black-and-white thinkers when it comes to musculoskeletal pain:

- "I can't see anything damaged on an MRI or X-ray."
- "There's no strong evidence on how to treat back pain."
- "It must be a 'soft tissue' injury (in other words, the medical system can't help you)."
- "Anti-inflammatories have the best evidence for short-term pain relief."

A good physiotherapist must train to understand everything about the body's movement that doctors do not, because we are the ones who work with the person, mentally and physically to put them back together and get them moving again. In many cases, there are too many variables to control to fully research the effectiveness of physiotherapy, because we use a variety of treatment tools that can be subtle and individual to the practitioner. We understand how the stability of individual ribs will affect your shoulder, how the stiffness in your hips will make you hinge in your back, or how the scar tissue from your C-section will restrict your movement. The biomechanics of the body are real, but they cannot be captured on an MRI, and doctors simply do not have the time to understand it. This is another reason why we have physiotherapists. Physiotherapy is a profession that should preach clinical mastery more than research-based practice, because human movement is not black and white.

Regardless, patients will likely still perceive doctors as the top of the medical hierarchy, especially "the specialist." People who have had pain for a long time tend to hold on to the notion that there is someone out there holding the key to their problems. A patient may have worked with their GP and a handful of allied health practitioners, but have to wait six months to see one special doctor, so they assume that the specialist must have the answer. In the pain world, these doctors are usually a physiatrist, a rheumatologist, an orthopedic surgeon, or an anesthesiology pain specialist. In my experience, once patients actually see their specialist, they are disappointed the vast majority of the time.

Physiatrists tend to do an assessment and write a report back to the GP, but this does little for the patient. Rheumatologists provide advice and, sometimes, an injection but are rarely game-changers. Orthopedic surgeons are experts at surgery, but once they have done their job, you shouldn't continue to count on them. Anesthesia pain doctors will perform nerve blocks and can seem like miracle workers one time and symptom-treaters the next. These doctors can be invaluable to the right patient, but I often emphasize to my clients to not get their hopes up, and not to sit around waiting in the medical model when there are plenty of "non-medical" therapies that might be better.

My key advice here is to be the leader of your own healthcare team. Research what you think is wrong with you, and keep your own healthcare record of what you experience and the healthcare workers who you have visited. Discuss with your friends and family who you should see, and build a team of allied health workers around you, including a physiotherapist, massage therapist, chiropractor, or naturopath. Go to your GP for problems you know they can help you with, but not with everything. Utilize different professionals' skills and judgments, and don't put blind faith in doctors. If you have to go through the medical system and wait for tests and appointments, remember that "the squeaky wheel gets the grease." Be polite, persistent, and sound a little desperate, and you will get through it faster and relatively unscathed.

# Diagnostic Testing:
# A Static Snapshot in Time
# of a Moving Being

X-rays, CT scans, and MRIs are useful tools when your doctor is trying to determine what is physically damaged or degenerated inside your body. They can give you tangible evidence of something physical that you can blame your pain on, but they often detract from the process of trying to determine why that structure is damaged.

A significant finding on a diagnostic test tends to stop the clinician's critical-thinking process required to push past what is injured and instead figure out why. This concept is particularly relevant in chronic pain issues that don't stem from a traumatic accident. It is also important in cases that began with a trauma, but where the person didn't heal or improve along the expected timeline.

An over-reliance of hands-off diagnostic testing is a fundamental reason why the medical model doesn't deal well with people suffering persistent pain issues, and it is why experienced manual therapists like physiotherapists and osteopaths speak a different language than doctors. Doctors will look at the pictures of inside your body, or they may just read the report that another doctor wrote about these pictures, and tell you what they believe to be wrong. A good manual therapist, however, will feel, watch, and experience your movements with you to better understand the movie that is happening in your body, instead of the snapshots of the aftermath. A significant finding on an MRI or EMG study can be a red herring and distract you from the true underlying problem.

A healthy body has good physiological movement in the joints, muscles, nerves, and organs. Tests that do not assess the body while vertical or during functional movements shouldn't be relied on too heavily to conclude what is or isn't wrong with a person. I have seen patients who move well and have no pain, but they have horrific-looking spinal X-rays, as well as people who are functionally crippled but nothing shows on their MRIs or EMGs. Medical tests should be taken into consideration after a proper and thorough physical exam has been performed, involving functional movements and skilled palpation (examination by touch).

The physiotherapist's skill set lies in understanding the interconnection between the skeletal, muscular, fascial, and visceral systems as they relate to movement. Not having the ability to freely order tests, inject painkillers, or prescribe medications has required physiotherapists to expand their tool box to understand and treat the body in a physical and conservative manner. Conversely, family physicians tend to lean on tests and medications and sometimes under appreciate the role of a physiotherapist working on the mobility of a specific rib to correct a shoulder problem or releasing fascia around the small intestine to decrease back pain. Manual therapy is a profession that lends itself more to clinical mastery than evidence-based practice, and this has, unfortunately, created a communication barrier between doctors and physiotherapists.

Evidence-based medicine suggests that doctors only utilize treatments that have the highest levels of evidence as proven by rigorous studies and clinical trials. It is a practice that makes sense and one that I support, but it is a process that is too black-and-white for the subtleties of physiotherapy. The physiotherapy approach to pain requires dealing more with the person, whereas the medical approach to pain tends to deal more with the symptoms and objective findings; sometimes you need one, sometimes you need the other, but usually you need both.

When I assess someone who has already had X-rays or an MRI, I prefer to put the reports aside and get a sense of how the person moves, functions, and feels before considering what the pictures say. X-rays largely look at bones only, MRIs visualize soft tissue, EMGs test nerve conductivity, and ultrasounds can show your organs, but there isn't a test that can evaluate how well your systems are or aren't working together. In many cases, the trained human eye and hands can provide a better sense of what is going on than a series of disconnected diagnostic tests.

You should take every diagnostic test related to your pain with a grain of salt; they can be helpful, but they can also be misleading. Consider placing more reliance in an experienced manual therapist to help you with your pain before trudging through the medical system with your discomfort. With physiotherapy, you will likely end up with a better understanding of why your body hurts and how you can deal with the pain conservatively, as opposed to medications, tests, injections, and surgeries.

# Phil the Pharmacist's Sore Back and Balls

Phil was a pharmacist who worked at a drug store near my office. He was about thirty years old, tall and skinny, and was more than frustrated with how much his back pain was disrupting his life. It had been going on for about six weeks by the time he saw me, and despite his best efforts, it seemed to be getting worse instead of better. He had seen his doctor, who ordered him an X-ray and CT scan, prescribed him anti-inflammatories, and referred him to physiotherapy. His X-ray was normal and his CT scan showed a mild bulging disc in his lower back. Phil found that the medication took the edge off his pain, but the physiotherapy exercises only aggravated his back and made it harder to work, so he came to see me on the recommendation of a family member.

Phil spent most of his workday standing and repeatedly bending to grab medications from the various cupboards in front of him. He was convinced that he had simply bent too far one day, and that was why his back continued to hurt. His doctor and previous physiotherapist seemed to agree, pointing their attention to the CT scan showing his L4/5 bulging disc. I was less convinced. I had seen many people with true disc herniations, and his posture, movement, and pattern of pain just didn't match what I was used to seeing. I didn't argue that he had a herniation, but I stressed to him that we shouldn't let it become a red herring.

Phil's skinny frame had a head-forward posture, rounded trunk, flat lower back, and tight hockey player hips. His posture needed some work, but his overall alignment wasn't that bad. I had him bend forward, backward, side to side, and stand on one leg, all of which he did reasonably well, but he could not, for the life of him, perform a squat by hinging in his hips. I demonstrated numerous times and gave him different cues, but the movement seemed impossible for his body. He was baffled in seeing me do what looked to be a relatively simple movement, but he could not find a way to make his body do it. I've seen "motor morons" (people who are baffled by simple movement exercises) struggle with the coordination of a squat, but he was an athlete, and it really seemed impossible for him. We both agreed that it was weird.

My first treatment of choice was to use intramuscular stimulation (IMS, or dry needling) to loosen up the muscles around his hips and lower back. He noticed an immediate freedom in his back that lessened his pain, but he still could not stand up and hinge in his hips without rounding his back. I let him go home and come back a week later to better gauge if the IMS had done the trick. He was a happy guy in that he had more improvement from a ten-minute IMS treatment than he did from his previous four weeks of physiotherapy exercises, but he still couldn't bend well and knew his back wasn't right. We did IMS three or four more times over the following month, which allowed him to work much more comfortably; still, we both agreed that there was something more contributing to his problem.

As it happened, I was starting my journey down the path of learning what is called visceral manipulation—a form of osteopathic manual therapy used to treat the mobility of internal organs. I was a relative master of IMS and quite proficient at movement and postural training, but I was a complete newbie with visceral work. Phil was a perfect example of why I was intrigued to learn more about this technique. It seemed to be worthwhile in trying when something just seemed off. Most practitioners have a musculoskeletal model of pain and injury in their brains, but not everybody fits well into that. While you can usually treat the muscles and joints to make a change, there is not always a profound treatment that lasts. In my experience working with mentors like Diane Lee and local osteopaths, I realized that the strange and resistant pain cases typically involved the patient's organs in one way or another.

Having only completed the first-level abdomen course through the Barral Institute, I started palpating Phil's front instead of focusing on his back. He seemed to have a pull to one side around his duodenum, the tube that connects his stomach to his small intestine. I worked on releasing this pull and sent him home to see if he noticed any change. He came back a week later with a funny look in his eye. After a month of loosening his muscles and trying every conceivable way to teach him to squat with his hips, he strolled in and said, "Watch this," and proceeded to do three perfect squats with no trouble. His back was better but still uncomfortable, and he wanted to know what exactly I did, because something that seemed physically impossible last week was now effortless!

To be honest, I'm not sure exactly what I released in him, but it made me want to learn more, because I thought it was just as cool as he did. This was the first time he visited and didn't feel like he needed me to needle him, because his muscles hadn't been tensing all week. It appeared that his back and hip muscles were tightening in reaction to protect his visceral pull, so for the first month I had only been treating his symptoms and not the root cause of his issue.

Over the next month, I experimented more with his guts; some weeks I made him better, while others I made him worse. This went on until I referred him on to a local osteopath who specialized in visceral work. I pulled back to my specialties of IMS and movement training and let the osteopath work her magic. Phil noticed subjectively and I noticed objectively how much better he started feeling and moving after a few sessions.

We progressed Phil all the way back to playing light hockey games, and he disappeared from my caseload for almost a year. Eventually he returned with a new but similar problem: his back was acting up again, but now his testicles hurt as well—badly. He was worried because the doctors said it was a vascular issue, and surgery would likely be required to correct it. Given the history of his back issues, I assumed his visceral mobility problems in his abdomen must be linked to this new testicular pain. I worked on his abdomen and urged him to see the osteopath again if he was unsure about surgery. My treatment helped him, but the pain forced his hand to follow the doctor's suggestion, and he went ahead with the vascular surgery in his lower abdomen. I saw him a few weeks later, and his response even further convinced me to learn my visceral and vascular anatomy. His ball pain was a bit better, but his back pain was largely gone.

Tension and stickiness in the fascia around your organs can restrict blood flow to and from certain areas. His body must have been protecting restricted blood vessels by not allowing him to squat and compress his groin area. The osteopath's and my treatments likely improved blood flow to his abdomen, resulting in less-reactive muscle guarding, decreased pain, and better movement. The surgeons were capable of getting right into the vessels to free them up and created a more profound version of our conservative therapy. Helping his back pain was a side effect of their intervention, but it helped clarify mine.

Phil is a good example of someone with chronic back pain who happened to have a positive finding on a CT scan that likely had nothing to do with his pain. I'm sure there are many people out there with chronic issues that don't make sense, because their healthcare practitioners are focusing too much on the outer frame of the body and not considering its contents.

Phil required two physiotherapists, an osteopath, and a medical doctor to get to the bottom of his issue. I can't stress enough that if you are having resistant pain issues, be sure to seek help from different health disciplines, because we all look at the body in our own unique way. I have found the combination of IMS, visceral manipulation, and postural awareness exercises to be the most effective way to deal with pain issues, but I also have a network of therapists and doctors around me to whom I refer clients as well. An integrated team approach is always best, because no one can fix everything!

# Preventative Health: Creating and Managing Your Own Record

When was the last time you went to your doctor? Your dentist? Your physiotherapist?

Why did you go? What was wrong with you?

What did your health professional tell you?

What did you learn from the experience? Anything? Do you remember?

Your body is a complex structure with all sorts of things happening inside that you likely don't understand. It is easy to leave the care of your body to others who "know what they are talking about" and just do as you are told, but it is a dangerous habit to fall into. Too much dependence on busy healthcare practitioners can result in you getting lost in the shuffle of a strained medical system. Your doctors or physiotherapists may be compassionate and diligent professionals with your best interests at heart, but remember that they likely see ten to twenty people every day, and it is easy for your care to fall through the cracks.

The best way to make sure you are taken care of is to become the leader of your own healthcare team and to learn something about your body with every interaction with your doctor, physiotherapist, or trainer. Keep track of these health-related experiences over the years, making written notes every time you have an injury or pain. Write down every time you see your doctor and what you learned from the appointment. Write down the advice your naturopath gives you, so you can refer to it again in the future.

You should create your own health record, in your own words, of what you understand to be wrong with you and what you could do to get better and prevent the problem from surfacing again. Your health is a product of everything you have done up to this point, and it can be extremely helpful to have a personal record of the past. Your health professionals take notes each time you see them, so why shouldn't you? You likely have paper charts and digital files all over the city with details that you don't have access to. Wouldn't it be better if you kept one comprehensive chart about yourself that you could refer to and learn from?

There are now countless smartphone apps that make it easy for you to take pictures, make notes, or save audio recordings, all at the touch of a button in a device that fits in your pocket and travels with you everywhere. I suggest you find an app that works for you in order to create some structure around your own health and to facilitate the communication between your various providers. As healthcare professionals, we are very busy and have a wide choice as to which electronic medical record platform we use. It is unlikely that we all pick the same one and seamlessly communicate with each other; but as the patient, you can choose a program or system that works for you, acting as the glue that holds your network together.

It is very easy to feel lost when forced to wade through a large medical system to address your problems, but it is much easier to maintain a feeling of control if you have your own system in place to document your past and present. The empowerment that comes from becoming part of your team makes a huge difference in dealing with issues like chronic pain, because the insecurity of the unknown creates stress, anxiety and fear—and that just make everything worse.

There is also evidence that simply documenting a behavior can be enough to initiate a change or improvement. Creating some form of data about yourself, whether it is subjective or objective, is a good reflective tool to create awareness of your lifestyle. The ability to look back on a month of what you have or haven't done can provide the motivation to help you stay or become active and healthy. If you do get injured, depressed, or sick, it may also come in handy to have a baseline record of what was "normal" for you. Your life can be turned on its head in a split second by an accident or illness, and it can be a difficult mental road to find normalcy again; if you have created basic structure in your life by means of a personal health record, though, it can provide a baseline and help you monitor your progress.

I recommend tracking things such as the following (pick one to three points that are relevant to you):

- Daily exercise: What, how much, with who, why, how you felt after?

- Aches, pains and injuries: What hurt, why do you think it hurts, what did you do about it?

- Visits to healthcare professionals: Why you went, who you saw, what you learned?

- Eating habits: When you ate, what you ate, why you ate?

- Personal goals: What are your goals, how are you going to meet them each month?

- Medications: What are you taking and why?

Evernote is my favorite phone and computer application for keeping track of all the information that comes at me in life. I encourage my clients to use their smartphones more to help them manage their health. Many aging adults still only use their smartphones as a calendar and a phone, but there is a whole world of applications they would greatly benefit from using. If you haven't been to the app store on your phone lately, spend some time browsing for simple tools that can help you keep your health in order.

# The Doctor with Knee Pain
# Who Didn't Believe Me

Dave the doctor was in the final year of his residency in internal medicine when I first met him. He was an avid skier and had recently taken up running to stay in shape while he was working long hours at the hospital. By the time he came in to see me, his knee had been bothering him for five weeks or so. He tried his best to deal with it himself by cutting down on running and taking anti-inflammatories, but it just wasn't doing the trick. He came in, open-minded, to try physiotherapy for the first time since he had become a doctor.

Dave's right knee hurt around his kneecap after about fifteen to twenty minutes of running. When it was flared up, he felt pain and had a hard time going up and down stairs or squatting up and down out of a chair. It felt better when he rested, but as soon as he started running again the pain came right back. He had accurately diagnosed himself with patellofemoral syndrome, but that only provided him with a name for his pain and not an explanation or a fix.

I explained to him that his knee pain was most likely a result of the tightness in his hips. I walked him through the anatomy and biomechanics of how the muscular and fascial tension from the deep muscles of his right hip were causing his iliotibial (IT) band to tug his kneecap laterally as he ran, which was creating friction and pain around the front of the knee due to poor tracking of his kneecap. He quietly listened and showed me a few times right where it hurt as he squatted down, but he seemed to understand what I was saying.

I then explained that the best way to fix his knee pain was to perform IMS, or intramuscular stimulation, an anatomy-specific form of acupuncture to help loosen the tense muscles in the leg and improve the biomechanics of the kneecap. Dave seemed to trust me, because I confidently answered all of his questions; so he agreed to the IMS, but he had plenty of questions about how the treatment was different from acupuncture, what was the mechanism behind IMS, what did the research say, and so on. I answered everything he asked as I treated his knee, making him squirm on the table with the deep crampy feeling of the needle in his hip.

After ten solid minutes of treatment while I explained and he grimaced while questioning, I finished what I needed to do and told him to get up and test it out. He looked at me with a somewhat skeptical glance as he climbed off the bed and onto his feet, performing a couple of squats. Dave's wide eyes and confused face said it all, but he looked at me while continuing to squat and said genuinely, "To be honest, I didn't believe you, but my knee doesn't hurt anymore. That's amazing, what did you call this again?"

I find treating doctors to be a unique challenge, because they typically believe they know more than they actually do about how the body works, and they are critical of anything that they haven't heard of before. I appreciate critical thinkers, though, and enjoy it when intelligent people wade into my area of expertise. I told Dave that the treatment is called intramuscular stimulation, and that you have to be a physiotherapist or a physician to use it. I gave him some reading material on the technique and told him to go for a run to test it out in the next couple of days.

I didn't see Dave again for quite a while, but I started receiving an influx of clients who were resident physicians at Vancouver General Hospital, so I knew he must have believed in me, because he referred his colleagues. He did return a few months later, though, this time with a different pain that he couldn't quite figure out; it didn't stop him from speculating, though. He was feeling a pain in his lower-right abdomen without any particular pattern of irritation. It didn't make sense to him, an internal medicine physician with pain in his abdomen. I examined him and discovered that his lower trunk was torsioned into an awkward alignment. I told him that I thought the twist in his lower thoracic spine was annoying the nerve roots of his upper lumbar spine, and that was referring pain into his abdomen. I thought he gave me a skeptical look with the explanation of his knee problem, but this time the skeptical look was much worse.

By this point, I had fixed his knee as well as the backs of several of his friends, so he went along with it again. I officially won him over by needling the muscles on either side of his thoracic spine to make his lower abdominal pain disappear. It took a few sessions to keep it away, but he started to consider the human body somewhat differently after his own experience in physiotherapy. He recognized that what he and many of his peers had brushed over in the musculoskeletal unit during medical school may have more to it, and that physiotherapists may have more expertise than doctors in this area.

# Why Knees Hurt

Your knees are simply big hinge joints that are built to flex and extend. together by four major ligaments called your MCL, LCL, ACL and PCL. ⌐⌐⌐ the middle of the joints are two C-shaped cartilage cups called your medial and lateral meniscus; these act as both shock absorbers and stabilizers. On the front of the joint, the kneecap functions to protect your knee and act as a lever to help strengthen the pull of your thigh muscles.

When I assess people complaining of knee pain, my first goal is to determine if one of the above-mentioned structures is physically damaged, or whether something is disturbing the mechanics of the joint, creating friction and causing pain; I estimate that 90% of the time it is the latter. Your knees and the structures that hold them together allow you to bend and straighten your legs freely, but they really don't appreciate twisting or torquing forces, which put your knees at the mercy of your hips and ankles. These joints are built to move in a variety of planes, but are prone to either tightening up or becoming weak, both of which result in negative effects on your knees.

The most common "diagnosis" of generalized knee pain is patellofemoral syndrome (PFS). PFS is not an ailment you catch like a virus or a cold, it is simply a name given to pain around the front of the knee. It typically arises when muscle imbalances in your hip and thigh disturb the mechanics of how your kneecap slides as you bend your knee. The poor mechanics of the kneecap create friction as you move that can eventually lead to pain and sometimes swelling.

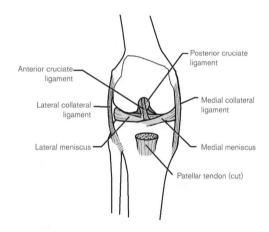

The kneecap pain is a symptom of something that is going wrong, so if you want to get rid of it you have to investigate why your hip and thigh muscles may have an imbalance. The answer is usually hidden in how your foot and hip are working together to load your leg in a stable manner as you walk or run. If your leg mechanics are quite good, the knee pain may even arise from a disconnect in how well your trunk muscles are working to coordinate your upper body with your lower body as you move. In other words, your knee pain may be resulting from any or all of the following: weak feet, tight calves, tight hips, poor alignment, a braced back, or poor core control. If you truly want to get rid of the problem, I would encourage you to look deeper than just icing your knee and getting orthotics; a good physiotherapist is the place to start.

...e absence of an acute injury, most knee pains develop as the manifestation of something that you do poorly on a regular basis. It may be how you stand or sit at work all day. It may be the funny position you sleep all night. It may be how you walk in the shoes that you have chosen. A physiotherapist can help loosen you up and correct your alignment, but when the root cause is something that you are unknowingly doing, you have to learn how to change the poor habit. Do you have a healthy posture? How do you sit at work all day? Are your cushy, supportive shoes really your best choice?

Sometimes knees do become structurally damaged. Plant-and-twist movements can result in the tearing of your meniscus or ACL (anterior cruciate ligament). If you tear your meniscus, the knee will usually subtly swell up over a couple days. It can be painful to bear weight on it, or it may produce intermittent sharp pains and even a feeling of locking. What you experience will greatly depend on the nature and location of the tear. A good physiotherapist or sports medicine doctor should be able to diagnose it for you. If you managed to tear your ACL, you may have heard a pop sound and the knee will have likely swollen up immediately. The knee will feel unstable, and your hamstrings will likely spasm to brace the joint. When enough torque is put on the knee, it is quite common to tear both the ACL and the meniscus at the same time.

**What should you do to manage knee pain?**

1. RICE: Rest, ice, compress, elevate.

2. See a physiotherapist for proper assessment, diagnosis and treatment.

3. Suspected torn meniscus?

   - Continue with physiotherapy and exercises. If it is not responding well after a few months, request an MRI from your doctor.

   - If the MRI confirms a tear, continue physiotherapy for up to a year.

   - If the problem persists up to nine months, pursue a referral to an orthopedic surgeon for a scope.

   - Rehabilitation from the scope surgery is about six weeks (you can walk that day, though).

4. Suspected torn ACL?

   - Continue physiotherapy and discuss need for a brace.

   - See family doctor about an MRI and referral to an orthopedic surgeon.

   - If you are young and active: Get surgery!

   - If you are older and more sedentary, continue with physiotherapy and try to avoid surgery. Your knee can function without an ACL and sometimes the joint will stiffen up enough to make surgery unnecessary for non-athletes.

   - Rehabilitation from surgery is six to twelve months.

Other common structural injuries are MCL sprains and dislocated kneecaps. These are the result of direct blows and require immobilization for up to six weeks. You should talk to your doctor and physiotherapist about the best brace to wear during the first couple of months. MCL braces will allow some flexion and extension, but dislocated kneecaps typically require the leg to stay straight for a month or so. These injuries are not generally repaired by surgery, so it is important to allow your body to create scar tissue for stability, and then work to regain the movement and function after four to six weeks. A physiotherapist will help you rebuild your strength and to identify all your compensation patterns from wearing a brace for so long.

Whether your knee pain arose as a biomechanical issue or due to a direct trauma, the eventual result can be osteoarthritis (OA). Poor mechanics over time lead to wear and tear, and the joint can slowly break down; pain is part of this process. Injuries that create instability, and surgeries that remove parts of your knee, may also lead to OA. Arthritis is effectively a structural issue in the knee. The cartilage wears off, small osteophytes grow, and fine cracks in the underlying bone cause the joint to slowly seize up. The knee will become much less tolerant to higher-impact activities, because the shock absorbers have worn out.

The best way to approach knee OA is activity modification and regular maintenance to the muscles around your hip and knee. The pain and irritation caused by the structural damage inside your knee will force the surrounding muscles to tense and can result in more unnecessary pain. I have enabled many people with horrific-looking knee X-rays to keep playing tennis at a high level simply by doing intramuscular stimulation (IMS) to their hips and thighs every four weeks. Having muscular tension released every month and ensuring you keep your legs as strong as possible will stave off an inevitable total knee replacement.

No matter how or why your knee hurts, the best approach you can take is to put your knee in a healthy environment by looking at your body as a whole and not only focusing on your sore knee. Make sure you have good alignment and learn to move well, and most knee pain will take care of itself.

# Allied Healthcare: Your Options Outside of the Medical Model

Most people are familiar with the medical model. You get hurt or sick, so you check in with your family doctor, walk-in clinic, or even the hospital to hear the doctor's opinion about what you have done. When it comes to illness and major trauma, a physician is definitely the one you want looking after you, but when it comes to pain, injury, and preventative health, both physical and cognitive, doctors are not necessarily your best choice. The fact that you even have a choice comes as a surprise to many people; most are under the assumption that their doctors know best. If you live in a moderate-sized city, chances are good that you can choose from a variety of allied health workers who have exceedingly more specialized training in physical health and rehabilitation than any doctor you will visit.

This passage includes a brief summary of common allied health professionals and the treatment options that they provide:

- Physiotherapist
- Massage therapist
- Chiropractor
- Naturopath
- Osteopath
- Kinesiologist/Personal trainer
- Yoga/Pilates instructor
- Counselor/psychologist
- Occupational therapist
- Traditional Chinese medicine/acupuncturist

Full disclosure: If you are not already aware, I am a physiotherapist and am moderately biased toward my own profession, but I do work closely and share clients with almost all of the different disciplines listed above.

**Physiotherapy, AKA Physical Therapy**

Physiotherapists (in Canada) are considered primary caregivers, which means you do not require a doctor's referral to see them. They now have a minimum of six years of university education and typically possess extensive post-graduate training in various specialties. Physiotherapy is a profession with a broad scope of practice which allows its practitioners to take the best techniques from many other healthcare disciplines and make them their own. I, for example, in addition to my kinesiology and physiotherapy degrees, attained diplomas in manual and manipulative therapy (this overlaps with chiropractic work), intramuscular stimulation (overlapping with acupuncture), as well as my extensive work in movement and muscle balancing (which overlaps with Pilates, yoga and coaching), and I have training in visceral (organ) manipulation (a manual technique borrowed from osteopathy). Some of my associates have specialized training in pelvic-floor work, cranio-sacral therapy, or even vestibular (inner ear) rehabilitation.

No physiotherapist is the same, because they have traveled so many paths in regards to specialized training. Their knowledge base, as mentioned, tends to overlap with physicians, kinesiologists, chiropractors, occupational therapists, massage therapists, Pilates instructors, osteopaths and acupuncturists, which can make them the links in a good healthcare team for a patient. While physiotherapists have the capacity to develop a very specialized skill set, their model of practice doesn't require their scope to become so compartmentalized as the medical model does for physicians. General doctors, like family physicians, don't have near as much training in musculoskeletal pain, and specialists often become too focused in their skill set to see the bigger picture when it comes to pain. Physiotherapists tend to fill in the gaps of service that doctors aren't able to provide; some doctors acknowledge this and some are blinded to it by how much they know and how entrenched they are in the medical model.

When choosing a physiotherapist, do your homework about who you decide to see instead of merely picking the clinic closest to your house. One physiotherapist may not be able to provide any relevant help, while another may change your life.

**Massage Therapy**

Massage has different meanings to different people, because there are many different types of massage techniques and massage practitioners. Sometimes it is used with the goal of relaxation, like in a spa setting, while other times it can be more goal-oriented and therapeutic—not to say that relaxation is not therapeutic. The various acts of using your hands to work on another person can often become grouped into the term "massage," because the discipline is more loosely regulated than a profession like physiotherapy; unfortunately, this can do a disservice to a group of highly trained and skilled manual therapists.

Many physicians and insurance companies do not adequately recognize the value a trained massage therapist can provide. Most registered massage therapists (RMTs) have extensive knowledge of muscular tissue, but there are other experienced therapists who possess specialized training in fascia (connective tissue), viscera (organs), cranio-sacral therapy (energetic connection of your skull to your sacrum), and what is called structural integration (Rolphing). Good RMTs blur the line between "massage" and osteopathy. I have worked closely with a number of them, and they all have a one-to-six-month waiting list; that must tell you they are doing something right, because believe me, most therapeutic manual therapy is not like a relaxing spa experience.

If you are looking for a good massage therapist, start by considering your needs and ask friends and other healthcare practitioners who they recommend. Look for people with specialized experience, and don't be scared off by a long wait to see them; it probably means they know what they are doing.


## Chiropractors

There is a general assumption that physiotherapists and chiropractors don't like each other, because they have different approaches and are somewhat competing for the same clients. I get asked all the time what I think about chiropractors. My short answer is: just like any profession, there are good ones and bad ones. I have treated many people who swear by their chiropractor and I have treated others who have been hurt by them. For my long answer, please see my article on WhyThingsHurt.com and read the lengthy discussions in the comments section.

I have worked closely with a few chiropractors and have taken some courses with others. I think a well-trained and experienced chiropractor can be an invaluable asset to a team. In practice, I don't refer my clients to them, but I am happy to work with them, because our skill sets complement each other more than they counteract. Their bread and butter is typically spinal adjustments, but many chiropractors will also offer active release technique (ART, a muscle stretch/release) or spinal decompression (a fancy traction table).

As I have suggested with physiotherapists and RMTs, do your homework when choosing a chiropractor, and challenge them if they are asking you to visit more than three times per week or to prepay for your appointments—sometimes business can get in the way of ethical care.


## Naturopaths

Naturopathic physicians understand the body in a way that medical physicians don't. I would never try to replace one with the other, but if your interest lies more in preventative health, I would consider adding occasional visits to a naturopath as part of your healthcare team. They better understand the role of stress and diet on the body and can use blood markers to evaluate health instead of disease alone.

In my experience, naturopath's common treatments involve recommending (selling) supplements, nutritional advice, IV pushes of supplements directly into your blood stream, prolotherapy (a sugar-based injection into soft tissues), acupuncture, and sometimes visceral manipulation. Their scope overlaps with medical doctors, holistic nutritionists, traditional Chinese medicine, and osteopathy. They provide a great service and can help you in ways you didn't realize, or they may hold the answer to issues you thought you just had to live with. My only caution or concern is how costly their visits can be if you don't have good insurance coverage. The recommended supplements they will sell you can get expensive quickly, but the overall service is a valuable one.

## Osteopathy

Osteopathy is effectively manual medicine. It is a discipline that has different recognition in different parts of the world. In my experience, it seems to be more commonplace in Europe and the eastern side of North America, but it is becoming more accepted and practiced by various manual therapists around the world. Osteopaths use their hands to manipulate the body to treat all of the different systems, including the bones, organs, nerves, muscles, and blood vessels, as well as the interaction between the systems. They are the originators of visceral manipulation, cranio-sacral therapy, spinal adjustments, and other manual techniques. Osteopaths' scope, as manual therapists, goes beyond musculoskeletal pain; their foundation is that a healthy body is one that has physiologic motion and mobility in all of the systems. They have developed precise and specific hands-on techniques based on an in-depth knowledge of functional anatomy.

As a physiotherapist, I have worked with a few therapists who are also trained as osteopaths, and they are always the ones I send my clients to if they plateau after working with me. Their skill set to treat obscure and resistant pain issues continues to fascinate me to the point that I am starting the training myself. Your location in the world will affect your ability to find a good osteopath. I know a number in Vancouver who started as physiotherapists or massage therapists and may still be working under that title. Many of them have such a devout following that it can take months to see them, but as I continue to suggest, do your homework and find the right match for you.

## Kinesiologists and Personal Trainers

The fitness industry is the most unregulated of all of the healthcare fields in that there is a huge variety in the education level of the person you may end up working with. In a personal training gym, you may find someone with a Bachelor of Kinesiology, a

Masters in Exercise Physiology, and a Certified Strength & Conditioning Specialist (CSCS) designation working alongside an uneducated but well-intentioned person who decided to do the basic-trainer certification through the local community center—and everyone in-between. Don't get me wrong, a well-intentioned person who safely motivates an inactive person into moving and becoming fit is an asset, but if you have lofty goals or special needs for your body, you should research the credentials of the person you are paying to whip you into shape.

If you are concerned about hurting yourself or need help rehabilitating from an injury to get back into the gym, I would look for someone with a kinesiology degree who has some affiliation with a physiotherapist.

If you want to train as an endurance athlete (a runner, biker, or triathlete), I would lean toward someone with a Masters degree or a CSEP (exercise physiology) certification.

If you are looking for high-performance strength training for sports and general conditioning, I would suggest finding a trainer with their CSCS certification, because their knowledge level and competency on form is that much better.

If you are trying to get back into shape after pregnancy, please don't jump right into "baby boot camp." I would advise to start with a screening by a physiotherapist, followed by a progression/combination of Pilates and kinesiology before pushing yourself too hard. At my clinic, we have set up an integrated program for postpartum women that includes a screening by a pelvic-floor physiotherapist, one-on-one clinical Pilates and kinesiology with progression to fitness.

Finally, if your goal is simply to become motivated into getting in shape, I recommend searching for a good personality fit over specific credentials. You want to make sure the person is competent, but the psychology of fitness training is hugely important. If you are going to be successful, you want to work with someone you respect and can learn from.

## Yoga and Pilates Instructors

The same applies for yoga and Pilates instructors as it does for kinesiologists and trainers: there are multiple certifications, little regulation, and a wide variety of knowledge levels. There are also many different types of yoga and Pilates, so do your homework before signing up for a class. If you are considering choosing either of them, I would strongly suggest starting with one-on-one sessions with an experienced instructor before you join a large group setting. There are nuances of body awareness that instructors can teach you which you just won't get out of group classes; once you go into them armed with the one-on-one experience, you will enjoy the classes more and be less likely to hurt yourself.

I refer clients to Pilates who need to develop movement awareness and abdominal recruitment with a certain degree of specificity. I find that Pilates helps people connect and relate to their bodies in ways that they didn't previously understand and that their time spent on developing body awareness makes my job easier in helping them to improve their posture. Although yoga and Pilates overlap in what they provide, I see Pilates as the journey and yoga as the destination. Pilates is more movement-based and yoga is more about holding a series of postures that target global flexibility and strength. Some people need to work on global flexibility and others benefit more from specific control exercises. One is not better than the other, it just depends on what you are trying to get out of it.

## Counselors and Psychologists

As a physiotherapist dealing with clients in various degrees of pain and discomfort, I have no choice but to be part-counselor at times. People, in general, will seek help more readily for a physical problem than a cognitive one, but, unfortunately, the two cannot be easily separated. Quite often a person will experience recurrent and persistent pains with strong ties to stress, tension, and anxiety, but the person is only willing to address the physical manifestation of their cognitive issues and wonder why the pain keeps returning. I encourage people to develop self-awareness both physically and cognitively, and counselors are the best professionals to guide this process.

## Occupational Therapists

I trained alongside occupational therapists (OTs) and have worked with them for thirteen years, but I still have trouble defining what exactly they do, because their scope is so broad. They tend to help people find the right assistive devices, make adaptations to their home, and learn techniques to compensate for physical and cognitive deficiencies after trauma or from aging. They tend to work in hospitals and the community in a way that overlaps with physiotherapists, social workers, and speech-language pathologists. If you, or a loved one, are having difficulty with activities of daily living due to a physical or cognitive deficit and need help to solve the situation, your best bet is to work with an OT.

## Traditional Chinese Medicine and Acupuncture

Traditional Chinese medicine (TCM) is an area which I don't have a great deal of experience or knowledge, so I will keep this short. As a healthcare provider, I have come to realize that not everything works for everybody, but some things work very well for certain individuals; TCM and acupuncture fall into this category for me. I respect anything that has survived the test of time over thousands of years and acknowledge that acupuncture is the foundation that intramuscular stimulation was built on—a tool that I use every day. TCM doctors are helpful when you feel that your body systems aren't working well together and need balancing. You may have trouble sleeping, allergies, pain, cancer, or just vaguely feel off. Acupuncture and other TCM practices can help subtly restore a homeostatic balance in your complicated, interconnected body.

## Conclusion

No single person knows everything when it comes to health, so be prepared to build a team of healthcare professionals around you, of which you are the leader. Be wary of practitioners who dissuade you from consulting others, and be open to treatment options that you didn't know existed. Do your homework and find professionals who are good for you, rather than ones who are conveniently located. Finally, keep track of your own health. Write down what you feel, who you see, and what they have told you. I promise, this information will come in handy again someday.

# Take Aways and Resources

**Take Aways:**

→ Doctors are awesome, but they may not always be your best choice or the most educated professional to help you with your specific problem.

→ X-rays, CTs, and MRIs only show structural issues, but many times the problem is movement-based and more related to how things are connected than how badly things have degenerated.

→ You can always have surgery, but you can never undo it. Pursue multiple different conservative treatments before going under the knife.

→ Be more assertive at keeping records of your own health.

→ Physiotherapists, massage therapists, chiropractors, naturopaths, osteopaths, and kinesiologists are all valuable healthcare professionals who you should consider in conjunction with, and sometimes instead of, your family doctor.

**Websites:**

✦ Evernote.com: a great application for your phone and computer to help you keep track of your life and health.

✦ IAHP.com (International Alliance of Healthcare Practitioners): a place to search for health professionals around the world by skill set.

# Why Things Hurt

## Myths to Dispel:

- Time heals all wounds
- Chronic pain has one root cause
- You didn't do anything wrong

# My Journey with Pain, Injury, Healing, and Understanding

I grew up in an active household as the son of two PE teachers. My dad always seemed to have a bad knee and my mom always seemed to have bad feet, but it never stopped us from getting out there. We all played sports and we all got hurt, but I seemed to have a special knack for it.

I still remember being excited for my first day of soccer as a five-year-old. The first practice was in the gym of a community center near our house. I walked down a long corridor and turned right to take a big step into the gym, ready to run around, but before I could take my second step, a soccer ball came out of nowhere to hit me hard in the face. My introduction to organized sports only lasted that one step, because I outright refused to go back and play there that year, but I later shook it off and went on to play competitive soccer for most of the next twenty-five years, relatively unscathed.

I was always one of the tallest and skinniest kids in my class, a collection of limbs that I managed to coordinate most of the time. I was perpetually one of the best athletes on my teams, but never the best, because I enjoyed playing all sports and never focused on just one. I struggled with aches as pains in my knees and Achilles tendons, because I was growing so fast while constantly running around, but it rarely stopped me because the fun trumped the temporary pain. Unfortunately, in grade seven, I had my first injury that really introduced me to the medical system.

I was pretty good at track and field as a ten- to thirteen-year-old, before all the boys started to hit puberty and develop real muscles. I regularly won provincial gold medals in high jump, long jump, and triple jump because of my build and good coaching, but none of that helped when I landed head-first on the gym floor in high jump practice. Five boys were practicing approaching the bar from the right side, and I was the only one jumping from the left, so each time they jumped the mat slid a few inches to the left—away from where I needed it to be. I ran up to the bar, jumped as high as I could, flopping over backward, but instead of landing on my shoulders on a soft, cushioned mat, I landed hard on the back of my head on the gym floor. I proceeded to throw up in the nurse's office, my doctor's office, and in the CT-scan machine at the children's hospital, where I stayed for the next three days as my world spun around me with a nasty concussion.

At thirteen, my invincible powers were still strong and I shook off the concussion to get back to my regular soccer and baseball games, but it wasn't long before I managed to hurt something else. Just over a year later, I was playing baseball and decided to try and steal third base. I corralled my lanky body into a full sprint and slid feet-first into the base, but as my luck had it, there happened to be a small rut in front of the bag that caught my right foot, and my momentum caused me to over-flex my knee and jam it hard into the ground. It hurt and I was called out, thankfully, because my knee swelled right up and was painful to walk on. I proceeded to ice it and rest on the couch for a few days, but when it just didn't improve my dad took me to the hospital. I don't think they found anything at the time, but the standard of care in 1990 was to put me in a full leg cast for two weeks with no follow up or physiotherapy. That knee still bothers me to this day.

My leg got stronger and I still managed to water ski, play soccer, basketball, and rugby that year, until baseball season came around again. Some mysterious force did not want me playing baseball anymore, because almost a year to the day, I ended up having the bones of my left forearm reset and casted after sliding into third base again. I sat on the bench for two innings and then walked home in pain before my dad took me to the hospital. It took three doctors and a lot of screaming to realign my bones, but six weeks in a cast seemed to fix it up pretty well, although, in hindsight, I'm sure physiotherapy would have helped my recovery.

High school involved a lot of rugby, basketball, soccer, and roller hockey, each coming with their own bumps and bruises, but the next significant incident happened when I was sixteen. My knee kept developing a bursitis while I was on a rugby tour in Australia, the summer after grade ten. It didn't hurt much, but I had a doctor in Queensland look at it, who decided to drain the swelling with a needle. It seemed to work like a charm at the time, but six months later my knee randomly turned red and became swollen and painful for no particular reason, to the point I couldn't put any weight on it. It felt like there were shards of broken glass inside my joint every time I put my foot down, so this time my sister got the honors of driving me to the hospital, where I endured the excruciating experience of having the ER doctor twice try to extract fluid from my knee joint with a long needle. It turns out I had a staph infection inside my joint, and I ended up staying in the hospital for three days on IV antibiotics.

It was business as usual once the infection calmed down, and I returned quickly to high school rugby. In my senior year, our team was ranked number one in the province and we had plans to go on another tour to Australia, New Zealand, and Fiji that July. At eighteen, I was six-foot-two and one hundred and seventy pounds soaking wet. I was pretty fast and pretty strong, but I had a body type more suited to swimming or volleyball than rugby. Two months before our provincial tournament, my shoulder decided that it would go with the two-hundred-pound Scottish kid who I tried to tackle instead of stay with me where I liked it. It was a dislocated shoulder, meaning the beginning of the end to my rugby career. Still feeling invincible, I rehabbed it for six weeks and tried to play again before the playoffs, but I only lasted two games before doing it again and was forced to sit on the sidelines and watch our team come in third place. I still went on the tour to the South Pacific with my buddies as a glorified water boy, which was an amazing experience but also a psychological challenge.

My shoulder was never the same after those two rugby games, and I managed to pop it out again while weight lifting, playing hockey, and rock climbing before I decided it was time to have surgery as a twenty-one-year-old kinesiology student. The surgery came at a time when I was just starting to apply for physiotherapy school. After six weeks in a sling, I ended up with a frozen shoulder that required my physiotherapist to tortuously manipulate to get it moving again. I was dedicated to my shoulder exercises and grilled my physiotherapist with questions about the interview process, and I ended up achieving success on both fronts: my shoulder started moving, and I got into all three schools that I applied.

In the last weeks of August, before I was to drive across Canada to attend physiotherapy school, I was wakeboarding at our family cabin in central British Columbia. Our wealthy dentist neighbor had just bought a top-of-the-line wakeboarding boat to pull his teenage daughters around the lake, but they were afraid of the big wake, so he enjoyed taking me out every so often. I was a good-enough wakeboarder to have the capacity to really hurt myself—a bad combination of skill and experience with no formal training. I entertained the crowd with my big jumps, until I tried landing a back flip; it felt like I broke my ankle and got punched in the face at the same time. Water can be a pretty hard surface to land on if you hit it awkwardly and with enough speed. Thankfully, my X-ray came back negative, but I had a nicely swollen ankle for my four-day road trip and started physiotherapy school armed with empathy for people in pain.

After that ankle injury, I actually strung together almost seven years without a substantial injury, even though I was playing soccer, hockey, and squash on a regular basis. I was now a physiotherapist with my own business in a personal training gym, my wife was pregnant, and I was trying to build my practice. Life was good, until one day while working with a client, I bent over the wrong way to pick up a light IKEA chair and ended up buckling to my knees and resting my arms on the plinth. My concerned client asked if I was OK, and ran to grab my receptionist when she noticed the sweat on my forehead and the discomfort in my eyes. I crawled onto my table and could not get down for six hours until I was drugged up and numbed with ice packs. I had tweaked my back before, but this time I just couldn't move. A few personal trainers helped me to the car and my extremely pregnant wife had to wait on me for three days while I lay helpless on the floor. I gained an entirely new appreciation for the debilitating effects of acute lower-back pain, but, thankfully, I knew exactly what to do and was back on my feet and at work the next week—before the baby arrived.

Acute pain after an injury is understandable, but when a problem develops slowly over time, its origin and why it won't go away can be more difficult to wrap your brain around. In my teens and twenties, most of my pains had an understandable cause-effect relationship. I did something stupid, and then I paid the price for it for a period of time, but it seemed to stop working that way in my thirties. I started doing fewer stupid things, but I also began getting random pains, which was frustrating. My right knee started vaguely hurting as I ran up the stairs, and my right hip would ache at random.

Being a physiotherapist, I tried treating it myself and had colleagues work on the problems, but nothing seemed to help, so I stopped playing soccer for a while; my hip actually started to ache more!

I eventually had X-rays and MRIs taken of my right hip and knee, which discovered a lateral meniscus tear, right where my pain was, and a torn labrum in my hip, with bony changes, too. Given that my knee had bothered me for over a year and that the tear seemed to be right where it hurt, I agreed to have an arthroscopic surgery to try and correct it as a last-ditch effort. Unfortunately, it didn't help at all and I am now much more resistant to sending my clients with meniscus injuries for knee scopes. The hip surgery was a bigger ordeal that I wasn't sure I wanted to undergo, especially after the result with my knee, so I decided to try what I wanted to do physically and if I just couldn't manage it, I would go ahead with the hip surgery. I wanted to play squash, a physically demanding and athletic game, twice a week. I opted to ignore my knee soreness and see how my hip would do. To my surprise, my hip started feeling better after regular squash and worse if I had to take a few weeks off. The multidirectional leg strength that I was developing seemed to be more important than the pounding I was giving it, so I opted against hip surgery.

After having three kids in three years, running a business, and trying to keep my body working, I had finally found a mix of athletic exercise that both my body and mind enjoyed, and which my schedule permitted. Squash once a week, ball hockey once a week, and chase the kids around on the weekends. Just as I seemed to find the perfect balance, though, my world was flipped on its head once again. As it turns out, I did another stupid thing. I played ball hockey without any eye protection and took a direct shot to my right eye that started a cascade of procedures and surgeries to save my vision, leaving me bedridden for over three months. I go into detail on this saga in a later section, but of all my injuries, nothing has impacted me more than the loss of my vision and the complications surrounding it.

My journey has taught me to reflect on the past, live in the present, and consider the future in my choices about my body and my health. I have experienced some amazing highs and some horrible lows that have given me wisdom ahead of my years to share with my clients as a physiotherapist. I have learned that it is better to have a tumultuous relationship with your body than none at all, because every accident or injury is an opportunity to develop more awareness and connectedness to your physical self. Physical setbacks are a time to work on your emotional fortitude, allowing you to come out mentally stronger and more intelligent on the other side. If you find yourself physically helpless, the best thing you can do is learn how to take control cognitively and come to peace with your situation to move forward positively.

# Perspective and Perception: A Lesbian Comedian, an Obsessive Accountant, and a Grumpy Old Man

I have worked with thousands of clients in my role as a physiotherapist, but there are only a select few individuals who have made a lasting impression on me, both as a person and as a therapist. Some have incredible stories, some are remarkably irritating, and others are the most ordinary people you could possibly imagine. Of this pool of select clients, there are three individuals who stand out as examples of how powerful perception is on the experience of pain, and just how different people can be. Laura, Clint, and Frank are three very unique clients who came to me in three very different ways, but they all had almost the exact same pain when they walked in the door. This is the story of how I helped them navigate their journeys of getting their bodies back in working order, and why I learned a lesson on human nature along the way.

My physiotherapy clinic has two different locations. The main clinic is a large space on the second floor of an office building in a retail shopping area of central Vancouver. It has a nice waiting room with a receptionist like you would expect at a proper clinic. My other office is more of a satellite location within a large medical building attached to the biggest hospital in British Columbia. I have a single room down a long hallway in the back of a family practice office; there is a small couch in the hallway and some instructions provided on the closed door, but no receptionist on site. Parking is a bit of a nightmare and the busy lobby is full of wandering old people, healthcare workers, and medical students, all trying to be somewhere on time. It can be a flustering place for some people to navigate.

The instructions on my door clearly say in large, bold, red letters, "Treatment in Progress, Please Knock," but some people like to learn by experience, more than by reading. Enter Laura. I was sitting at my desk, just finishing up some charting after I had eaten lunch, but I still had about fifteen minutes to spare before I was expecting my first client for the afternoon. She made a very Kramer-like entrance into my office. Her unkempt brown wavy hair was everywhere. She was eating a very crumbly scone from Starbucks in one hand while holding its brown paper envelope in the other hand, as well as a bike helmet, a burlap bag, and her wallet. With her mouth full of scone, she dumped her belongings onto the chair and proceeded to lay on the floor and show me some movements that gave her pain, all before saying "hello," fifteen minutes before her appointment time, and eating her crumbly scone the entire time. Amazing! I was too blown away and amused by the situation to be annoyed.

Laura came to see me about her bad back. She didn't know what she had done, but her lower back seemed to cause her trouble while sitting in the car, rolling over in bed and bending over the sink to brush her teeth, as I learned in her very animated fashion within the first ninety seconds of our meeting. She was an amateur comedian-slash-unemployed forty-year-old lesbian with remarkably horrible fashion sense, and she was my new favorite person. She talked about her back pain in a nonchalant way, but I could tell it was impacting her life. She had tried massage, hated the gym, and had a friend suggest that she see me, but she hadn't inquired at all about what I do. Laura floated through life without much thought about direction or detail; she very much lived in the present.

Clint was the opposite. Everything Clint did was purposeful and controlled. He was a forty-year-old accountant with borderline obsessive-compulsive disorder. He had a government job and knew exactly what his benefits plan would and would not cover, so he pre-booked weekly sessions as far ahead as I opened my schedule to maximize his insurance plan. He spoke with a bit of a stammer, as if he was worried about every point and every question he ever had. He was a nice man, but his attention to detail was almost paralyzing for him. I'm sure he was a great accountant.

Clint also came to me about his back. He was having trouble sitting for the long hours his job required, and he would wake up every morning with stiffness, pain, and trouble straightening up. His massage therapist had suggested he try intramuscular stimulation (IMS) and more exercise, so he came in to see me after having researched both topics as well as my background. Clint hung on my every word and made sure to write down every last detail, because he needed to have everything just right.

Frank was a retired, seventy-four-year-old Portuguese man who had done physical labor most of his life, and he only came to see me because his wife was tired of listening to him complain about his back. He was the type of man who entrusted his health in the hands of his family physician and would do what he was told and nothing more. He was a hardened man of few words with a thick accent and even thicker skin. I tried to get a sense of how much his back was hurting on a scale of one to ten, and he replied in his thick Portuguese accent, "I had a radiator blow up in my face once, that hurt, so my back . . . my back, I will say it is a two." Pain is relative and Frank had been sucking it up for a long time.

I get a pretty good sense of a person and what may be wrong within the first five minutes of meeting. I pay attention to how they walk into the room, how they sit in the chair, how they tell me their story and especially how they take off their clothes. I end up building a funny relationship with people that involves them telling me their troubles while they get into various degrees of undress. Being a physiotherapist, I am somewhat numb to being exposed to strangers' partial nudity, but there are definitely different strokes for different folks. Laura removed her shirt and threw it on the floor in the corner of the room after she finished her scone and was ready to undergo treatment in her well-worn bra, baggy pants, and boots. Clint came to every appointment wearing the same shorts and T-shirt, folding his shirt neatly and placing it precisely on the chair. Frank took his sweet time to expose the smallest area of skin under his layers of tucked-in undershirts and button-up plaid shirts. I had to factor "old-guy change-time" into our thirty-minute appointments.

Laura told dry, witty jokes about her body the entire time I assessed her. She seemed comfortable and insecure at the same time, but was content to be in a place where she was dealing with her problem. Clint tried anxiously to help me with every movement I took him through and had a clarifying question for every single thing that I said. Frank, on the other hand, seemed to be part deaf and only half paying attention to the young guy who wasn't even a doctor. They all got through their first thirty minutes with me in their own way, and I managed to make a connection with each of them by listening and explaining their back pain in a context that made sense to them. Laura was interested in my explanation but was game to do whatever I said. Clint ate up every detail I said and would have talked about it for three hours if I let him, while Frank half-listened to me and half didn't care; he just wanted me to fix it and tell him what to do.

Each of them had a torsion in their pelvis due to an imbalance in their hip muscles, resulting in compression and irritation in their lower backs. Laura had it for five weeks, Clint had it for six months, and Frank had it for eight years. None of them attributed their pain to a particular accident or injury, but all had suffered, to a certain degree, with pain and dysfunction. I explained the biomechanics to each of them based on their level of interest. I explained that the best way to fix their problem was to use IMS, a form of dry needling similar but different to acupuncture. Laura's eyes bugged out of her head, Clint had even more questions, and I think Frank thought I was a quack, but I convinced all of them to give it a try.

I explain to people receiving IMS for the first time that they will have a love-hate relationship with the treatment. It is not the most comfortable procedure in the world, but it can seem like magic if it releases the right thing. It involves using an acupuncture needle to release taut bands of muscle deep in the hips and spine and can feel like a deep, crampy pressure for about five to ten seconds while the needle is inserted. (I go into full detail on the process and the theory of IMS in following chapters.) In order to free up Laura, Clint, and Frank, I needled both of their hips, the small of their back, and their inner thighs. The process took about ten minutes for each of them.

Laura became even more entertaining when she was nervous; she had plenty to say while she was lying on her side with a butt cheek hanging out of her grungy pants. The first point I typically release is the gluteus medius on the side of the hip, and it can pack a punch. It is a deep, strange sensation that most people don't know what to do with. Laura yelled really loudly, "Whoa, whoa, fuck, really, fuck, fuck . . . Oh thank God, is it out, is it out?" and then laughed hysterically. I'm pretty sure we gave her some material for her act. After she wrapped her brain around what the first few needles felt like, she calmed down and was totally fine. Once I told her that I was done, she stood up, sweating profusely, and walked around the room looking confused. She bent over to grab her shirt from the corner of the room and stood back up with her jaw hanging open. She asked if I was some sort of sadistic, voodoo healer genius, because her back now felt awesome.

Clint had questions up until the moment I tapped the first needle into his hip, and I discovered his off switch. He looked like he wanted to say something, but nothing came out. His body tensed and his mouth opened, but he was silent until I took the needle out and then he said, "What do you call this again? How is it different than acupuncture? Why are we needling down there, when my pain is over here?" and so on, until I stuck another needle in him and then . . . silence. I answered the questions that needed to be answered, but in order to get through our appointment on time, I had to cut him off with needles about eight times. When we were done, he stood up and felt like he had been hit by a truck. He was braced and stiff and looked very concerned. I assured him that post-treatment soreness can be normal, and that he may hate me today but will probably love me tomorrow. I sent him home to have a hot bath and to drink plenty of water.

Frank lay there stoically and didn't move, make a sound, or even change his facial expression the entire time. When we were done, he stood up and took ten minutes to put his pants back on, tuck in his shirts and say, "So, that is it? We are done?" He left barely saying two words to me, but I happened to treat his wife a few days later and she told me how fantastically better he was moving and feeling, so she made another appointment for him to return the following week.

Laura's, Clint's, and Frank's first experiences with IMS were very much reflections of their personalities. They all ended up with marked improvements from the treatment, but the filters through which they experienced it were much different. People ask me whether IMS hurts and I always say that it really depends on your body type and your personality. Some people experience little pain and others have to use their own coping mechanisms to deal with the discomfort. I have seen a two-hundred-and-fifty-pound man sooth himself by singing "Frère Jacques" quietly and old grannies drop F-bombs. Everybody is different, but most people can be helped if you find the way in for them.

Laura saw me once a week about three times until we eliminated the back pain from her daily radar. She had more physical issues which we could have worked on to help prevent recurrence of her issue, but Laura's personality of living in the present, combined with her unstable financial situation, made her time with me short. She gave me a good perspective on how different people have different relationships with their bodies. She hadn't lived a very physical life, she wasn't an athlete, and her previous experiences with pain were largely based on her being clumsy. Her back hurting didn't really keep her from doing her daily activities and she generally didn't worry about much so she was fairly lighthearted about the whole experience. Pain can dominate some people's lives and significantly impact their personality, but Laura was able to compartmentalize her experience and avoid fear, anxiety, and obsession related to her discomfort. A sense of humor can go a long way.

Clint was serious even when he was joking. I saw him fifty-two times over a couple years and couldn't convince him that treatment was no longer necessary. He returned a week later after our first session with his back feeling much better, after enduring two days of soreness and living on a heating pad. I think my telling him that his pelvis was misaligned put his obsessive mind into overdrive. He became focused on left-right differences in his body and little physical incidents that had happened to him over the years, to the point that his original back pain ceased to be the topic of concern after a month or two.

Clint, being Clint, and armed with a good government benefits package, would not be satisfied until he experienced no pain and his body was perfectly symmetrical. After needling him a few times, I talked to him about teaching him to move better, improving his posture, and getting stronger in order to prevent any future issues with his back, which he thought was a great idea. We shifted gears into movement training and developed an extensive repertoire of home exercises for him in a detailed binder with his annotations under all of my drawings. I regularly tried to give him exercises where he had to do seven repetitions on one side and ten on the other, or get him to just work on one side and not the other to mess with his obsessive-compulsiveness, but I never got away with it. Clint was my best student; he did everything I showed him, learned to move really well, and got quite strong, but he became obsessive about other pains and areas of soreness in his body to the point that I felt he just needed a break from everyone, including himself. I told him as much and tried my best to discharge him, but it took another three months before I was able to wean him away from me. Some people need to be encouraged to do and think more while others need to learn to do and think less. Clint needed to learn to distract himself from himself.

Frank returned two weeks later, as grumpy and skeptical as ever, but he didn't realize that I could tell more about how he was doing by watching him move than listening to what he said, or that his wife had ratted him out the previous week. He rose from his chair much faster and with greater ease, and he was standing much more upright as he complained to me that his back was feeling better for about five days before it worsened again. He told me that IMS doesn't last and that he was too old to be fixed. I clarified his complaint by explaining that most people with a twist in their pelvis experience about five days of relief from IMS before an element of it starts to return and that we would treat a little more each time and he would likely get a longer-and-longer-lasting result. I thought that five days of relief after eight years of pain may have impressed him, but he gave me nothing.

In Frank's second session I treated his hips and back like the first time, but also worked a bit on his mid back and neck, because eight years of being out of alignment had created a few torsions in him beyond his pelvis. I decided to not bother explaining it to him; instead I just fixed it and told him what to do like he wanted. He didn't say much, but his energy changed and he started asking about his next appointment. After four sessions in about a month, Frank's back started feeling pretty good and he started talking to me. It turned out that I knew what I was doing after all and I earned his trust.

His wife told me that he religiously did the three exercises I gave him and she started just making him appointments to see me once a month to help prevent his complaining from coming back and they were both happy. Frank was stoic in many ways, but needed to be shown that there are times to be stoic and there are times when you should just ask for help. Many men need to learn that toughing it out is not always the best option when it comes to their body and that they should at least put as much maintenance into their bodies as they put into their cars.

Laura, Clint and Frank are good examples of how different people approach and perceive the world differently, and how anxiety, fear, stubbornness, and humor can have an effect on pain management. It is probably the biggest reason why back pain is so difficult to study and to provide "strong evidence" for the various forms of treatment; the personality of both the patient and the practitioner can have a profound impact on the outcome of the therapy. There is an art and a science to being a good physical therapist, but it begins with being a good "people-person" and appreciating the crazy in everyone. Once you can wade through a person's idiosyncrasies and earn his or her trust, it is easier to assess and provide treatment objectively and properly.

# Chronic Pain: A Product of Integrated Systems

Every few years, it's important to challenge everything you believe to be true, either by learning something new or by trying to look at the same thing from a different angle and seeing what sticks. I have done this with physiotherapy, pain, and anatomy and have been blown away by how much my approach to the body has changed over the years. I started by learning through my kinesiology degree about muscles and how they attach to bones. I learned about how muscles contract and what nerves extend to what muscles; it was a lot to memorize at the time. When I entered physiotherapy school, I was able to see and touch real specimens in the anatomy lab (it sounds creepy, but it was great learning tool).

Physiotherapy school was broken into different units to help us learn about the various systems in the body. There was "neuro," where we learned about the nervous system, brain and spinal cord injuries, and neurological disorders. There was "cardioresp," where we learned about the lungs, the heart, and issues like cystic fibrosis, COPD and the basic physiology of how the body stays alive. Finally, there was "ortho," where we further discovered muscles, bones, ligaments, and tendons and all the things that may go wrong with them from a medical perspective. These units were compartmentalized in school, and, in hindsight, that was necessary to allow us to learn in just a few short years the vast amount of information there is to know about the body. As a physiotherapy student entering the workforce, I knew a little bit about a lot of things related to the human body, but relatively little about any one area. I had a foundation of knowledge that required experience to make it meaningful.

I was told by a few experienced physiotherapists that "you have to fake it till you make it." I'll never forget one of my first clients as a new graduate: he was a factory worker who got his pant leg caught in a steel drum press that pulled his leg in and crushed it until he saw it coming back at him in the wrong direction. A co-worker managed to hit the emergency stop button just in time to save him, but his leg was severely damaged. Doctors had managed to reconstruct it, and my job was to try and get it moving again and to have him attempt weight bearing on it; that man endured a lot of pain, but his rehabilitation was relatively straightforward compared to the types of people I see today.

Acute pain and chronic pain are different animals. Acute injuries require time, perseverance, and proper guidance to help people recover and restore optimal movement and function. Chronic pain requires detective work and a genuine understanding of how the different systems in the body play off each other in order to get it under control. It requires a practitioner to "decompartmentalize" what they have learned and look at the problem in a new way, a practice that physiotherapy is progressively improving on, and one which medicine is continuing to fail in. Medicine is very much a compartmentalized profession that accomplishes incredible things to save people's lives, but chronic pain crosses too many of its boundaries for it to be an effective solution to the problem.

Ongoing pain in the absence of a noxious stimulus can be the product of one or many systems in the body. The bony framework and the muscles that move it get blamed for far too much, because they are the most accessible systems. The nervous system is often next in line for blame as the electrical wiring of the body, but the visceral system is largely overlooked when it comes to pain. Your body is very protective of its organs, and when they don't move properly, you won't either. Fascia, as the connector and supporter of everything in the body, is a focus in a growing area of study; body workers have learned to appreciate it more and more in the recent years, as well as mindfulness—the impact of cognitive factors on the perception of pain.

All of the systems play a role in pain, but none more than the flow of blood through the vascular system. Body parts can't function without nerve input, but they can't survive without blood flow. The interconnection of these systems is astonishingly complex and endlessly fascinating for a budding anatomy nerd like myself. The more that I have departed from the medical model's view of pain, the more that I have learned to feel, listen, and treat the subtle systems in the body, and the more successful I have been at helping people with their chronic pain problems.

My first post-graduate series of courses focused on learning the detailed biomechanics and arthrokinematics of the bones and joints in the body; in other words, learning how to feel, move and manipulate spines, shoulders, hips, knees, ankles, elbows, and wrists. I developed a sense of touch that I didn't have before, but it was like someone giving me a thousand-piece puzzle with no picture on the box. As I finished the manual therapy program, I started working with and taking a series of courses from a physiotherapist named Diane Lee. Diane helped me develop a framework to look at the body as a whole, which helped me to make sense of all the pieces I had been given. She introduced me to the role of organs in pain and alignment issues, the concept of mindfulness, and the technique from Dr. Chan Gunn called intramuscular stimulation (IMS), all of which have made huge impacts on the path of my career.

In May of 2008, how I assessed and treated people fundamentally changed after learning how to use IMS from Dr. Chan Gunn near the end of his career. IMS allowed me to tap into a person's nervous system and, very specifically, turn down the volume in certain areas to calm the compressive muscular tension that was causing pain. The process of treating pain naturally taught me about the interconnections and referral patterns in the body that don't intuitively make sense. I started fixing things that I couldn't before. Having a background in manual therapy, the needle became an extension of my hand and allowed me to literally feel inside the muscles. To this day, it is still the most powerful technique I have ever learned.

After five years of honing my needling skills, I decided to further pursue my understanding of what I used to call Diane's "visceral voodoo," because I was noticing a subset of clients who didn't respond or receive a lasting result from IMS. I was fairly cynical about this light-touch form of manual therapy that supposedly allowed you to "listen" to the body with a light touch and feel for gentle fascial pulls coming from the organs. I saw Diane do it, and I didn't get it, but I trusted that she knew what she was talking about, so I signed up for a visceral manipulation program through the Barral Institute, a series of courses developed by French osteopath Jean-Pierre Barral. I am still going down this rabbit hole of learning the osteopathic approach to manual therapy, and it continues to intrigue, impress and fascinate me, all the while pushing me to take more courses in order to squash my flickering skepticism. I have learned a level of anatomy that I didn't know existed and have come to realize that there are galaxies of interconnections in the body that I am not ready to learn yet. Visceral and neural manipulation may appear hokey to some medical professionals, but it is strongly rooted in anatomy and hours of clinical expertise laying hands on people that many doctors don't understand.

Through the Barral Institute, I had the opportunity to participate in a fresh cadaver dissection course with a group of other physiotherapists, massage therapists, and osteopaths. Over three days we meticulously dissected two donors' bodies that had only just died within the week, and had never been frozen or preserved. It would be a horrifying experience for most people, but a fascinating one for healthcare professionals who seek to understand the intricate web of connections in the body as their means of conservative treatment. I had the opportunity to place my finger on a membrane in the skull while another person moved the donor's ankle and I could feel the tug all the way up in her head. I pulled on a small branch off the sciatic nerve in her calf and could see how much it tugged all the way up near her tailbone. We saw the after effects of numerous abdominal surgeries and even found and touched cancerous tissue, gallstones, and uterine fibroids. I believe that every health professional who pokes and prods people for a living should seek out the opportunity to experience how our bodies are held together by getting right in there and feeling it firsthand.

In only three to four years of learning and trying to integrate visceral and neural manipulation into my tool belt of techniques, I had truly gained an appreciation for just how connected the body really is. I've discovered that I can markedly free up a stubborn hip by manually releasing a membrane that attaches to a bone behind the ear. I figured out that old appendix scars can and will tighten a person's right ankle. I returned a lady's kidney function to normal range by releasing fascial restrictions in her abdomen as measured by three blood tests. I calmed down another lady's chronic left sciatica by releasing tension in the palate of her mouth. I, personally, have had my chronically high-arched, rigid feet substantially improve and relaxed by having my lungs and pericardium worked on. It blows me away and creates happy disbelief in my clients when I fix something in a very indirect way.

Sometimes things are straightforward and sometimes they are not. Many health practitioners, medical and allied, get confined by the commonly understood nerve referral patterns in the body, such as how leg pain comes from the lower back and arm pain comes from the neck. In many cases, the spine referral patterns hold true and are invaluable information, as demonstrated by the effectiveness of IMS. To be thorough, however, you need to take the assessment one or two steps further and ask what is irritating the spine enough to create this pain. Unfortunately, convention typically has most practitioners stop at what we can see on diagnostic tests like X-rays and MRIs, and the power of a trained hand is underestimated.

Our bodies are full of sensory feedback loops that cause us to experience the world with all of our systems. We deal with our emotions subconsciously with our mind and body. How you feel affects how your organs function and move, which, in turn, affects the mobility of your body. Stress, pain, anxiety, and fear affect your physiology, your flexibility, and your function.

Chronic pain has many layers that are an entangled mess of the physical and the emotional; in order to help a person recover, you need tools that can help you deal with both. Visceral manipulation is a manual technique that gives the practitioner an opportunity to treat the connection of the physical and the emotional. IMS allows the physiotherapist to calm your nervous system and relax your muscle tone, while the education of a client to practice mindfulness and body awareness is the glue that holds everything together.

If you are having chronic pain problems, I encourage you to find someone to help you who has the capacity to treat you as a whole person. Many healthcare professionals will treat the container and not the contents of the body. Your brain, organs and nervous system as a whole are typically the missing link to solving the pain puzzle. Depending on where you live, physiotherapists likely have the broadest scope of the tools you may need, but don't be afraid to utilize more than one healthcare professional, because no one can do everything. Research the people you see and be an advocate for you own well-being, rather than putting blind faith in your physician

The following is a schematic originally developed by Diane Lee and Linda-Joy Lee that represents all the different pieces of the puzzle healthcare professionals need to consider when dealing with a person in pain (see next page). The approach is called the Integrated Systems Model (ISM) and continues to evolve at Diane's lead. ISM has helped physiotherapists around the world make sense of chronic pain. The patient's story is at the center of a process that requires the therapist, by means of manual palpation and movement screening, to problem solve what is the root cause, or "driver," of the pain problem in the person's body. ISM creates structure for the process of determining if it is a joint, a nerve, an organ, or a muscle that is causing the problem and how the role of body awareness and emotional stress can impact everything. Diane champions the importance of clinical mastery while working on formal research to further validate this model; it is a path that I hope physiotherapy continues to follow.

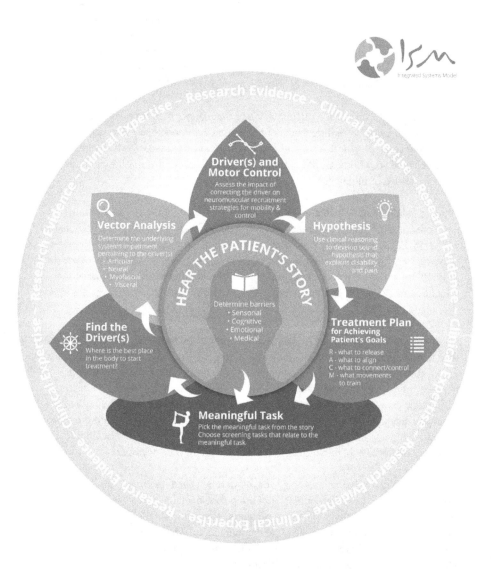

# Why Backs Hurt

If your back has ever "gone out" on you, you will appreciate the following section and may learn how to fix your nagging back issue. Back pain can take many forms and is, hands down, the most common issue that brings people into a physiotherapist's office.

- "It hurts when I bend over to brush my teeth."
- "I can only sit for ten minutes before I have to move."
- "Walking triggers a pain deep in my butt."
- "I bent forward and couldn't get back up."

It happens to the best of us. I have seen inactive, overweight people with back pain, insanely fit personal trainers with back pain, elite athletes, new moms, desk jockeys, and I have personally suffered from it on occasion. You can have the strongest core in the world and still be susceptible to hurting yourself or experiencing pain in or around your back. In this article I have outlined the most important factors as to why backs hurt, because back pain requires an explanation of what is going wrong as opposed to a diagnosis of a condition.

## Step 1 to understanding:

Things happen for a reason. You don't simply catch back pain like you catch a cold. It is usually related to something that you have done or are continuing to do poorly, like standing, sitting, walking, breathing, bending, or lifting. An accident or an acute injury can set pain into motion, but how you deal with the injury, pain, and mobility after the fact is the important part. You have to take ownership of your ailment and consciously work at improving your situation. You may need something loosened for you, you may need to learn to move more efficiently, you may need to lose weight or may even need surgery. In nearly every case I see, back pain can be made significantly better if addressed properly.

## Step 2 to understanding:

Back pain is rarely the result of one damaged structure that can be visualized on an X-ray or MRI. You may find that you have a bulging disc in your lower back, but if so, I would refer you to Step 1: "Things happen for a reason." Why do you have a bulging disc in your lower back? Discs bulge for a reason. The way you are moving or sitting is likely causing too much stress on your disc, so the answer shouldn't be "strengthen your core" or surgically fix the disc, but rather to learn what part of your body is making your disc work too hard and to figure out how to change it.

**Step 3 to understanding:**

Everything is connected more than you realize. Stiffness in your ankle from an old sprain may be causing you to compensate in your hip when you walk and may be throwing your back out of alignment. The fall on your hip three months ago that only hurt for a few hours may have damaged the mechanics of your hip and pelvis, and now your back hurts. The fact that you always lean on your left side in an L-shaped couch to watch TV may shift your rib cage and put uneven pressure on your lower back. These are the problems that are responsible for chronic lower-back pain—issues elsewhere in the body that have put the lower back in a bad environment.

An adept healthcare practitioner who can do a thorough physical assessment should be able to figure out the primary driver or root cause of your problem. I suggest finding a physiotherapist who will approach your care as a puzzle that needs solving, and not simply a symptom that needs treating.

**Step 4 to understanding:**

Lower-back pain is most commonly an interplay between the following:

- Your hips are either too tight or have more flexibility than you can control;
- You have a left/right asymmetry in the above hip issue, which is creating a twisting force on your pelvis;
- Your pelvis is the base where your lumbar spine sits, and when it is torsioned it will typically compress the lower vertebrae in your back;
- The compressed joints in your lower back annoy the nerves that innervate your hips/legs; and/or
- Your hips/legs become tight because the nerves in your back are annoyed.

And so you have started a vicious cycle:

- If your pelvis is twisted, a number of your ribs tend to shift to compensate;
- Your shoulder sits on your rib cage, and if your ribs are shifted, your shoulder might become sore;
- There are big muscles that attach your shoulder to your neck; and
- If your shoulder isn't working right, it is very easy to develop neck pain.

This entire process can start at the top and work down, in the middle and work outward, or at the bottom and work upward. The key to treating your back pain is figuring out the pattern.

Your lower back is likely the symptom and not the cause, regardless of what you see on an MRI.

**Step 5 to understanding:**

In order of importance, there are six factors to consider when evaluating your back pain:

1. Posture

2. Movement/biomechanics

3. Alignment

4. Strength-flexibility balance

5. History of injury

6. Structural damage or degeneration

Unfortunately, most people tend to focus on the above factors in reverse order. I have seen countless clients with horrific-looking X-rays and almost no pain. I have also seen people with perfect-looking X-rays and MRIs who continue to suffer. Diagnostic tests, for the most part, are static snapshots in time of your back and don't really tell you why backs hurt, only what is damaged.

**Step 6 to understanding:**

There are many systems in your body that make up who you are. Your skeleton forms your structural framework; your muscles support and move your skeleton; your organs keep all the systems alive and functioning; your fascia helps hold everything together; and your nervous system provides the electrical wiring to connect all of the systems. These integrated systems create a body that is built to move and think freely, but any or all of them have the capacity to limit normal movement and can create pain if something goes wrong.

The mobility of your fascial system is strongly affected by surgeries and scar tissue. The flexibility of your muscular system is contingent on the irritability of your nervous system. The irritability of your nervous system is equally affected by the health of your spine, as well as cognitive factors like stress and anxiety. Our ability to over-think problems can leave us out of touch with our bodies and in unnecessary pain. Simple tasks like how you sit, stand, breathe, and walk are hardwired into you from a young age, but have been affected by your injuries, jobs, sports, and behaviors. The key to fixing your lower-back pain is to assess which of your systems is causing the most problems with your daily tasks, and to try to change it.

**How to change:**

I tell my clients that I am going to guide them through the process of release, re-educate, rebuild. I explain to them that we are going to find the tight structures that are restricting their mobility and alignment, and we are going to try and release them (see a list of the release techniques, below). Releasing these tight, pulling structures will open a window to allow the person to move differently; this is when the client must gain some awareness of how their body feels different and practice some movements to re-educate the body for better movement patterns. Once good movement patterns are developed, it is time to build strength to reinforce them; this is how you create lasting change. Skipping the middle step and trying to build strength on top of dysfunction will bury the problem deeper and make the body more resistant to change.

Release techniques to try:

- IMS (intramuscular stimulation)
- Manual therapy (mobilizing or manipulating the joints)
- Visceral manipulation
- Neural manipulation and cranio-sacral therapy
- Myofascial release
- ART (active release technique)
- Structural integration
- Various types of massage
- Self massage using foam rollers, The Stick, release balls

Re-education techniques to try:

- WhyThingsHurt.com exercise videos
- Clinical Pilates in a one-on-one setting
- Yoga in a one-on-one setting
- The Feldenkrais method

Rebuild techniques to try:

- Qualified kinesiologist or strength and conditioning coach

# What is IMS Acupuncture? IMS vs. Traditional Chinese Acupuncture

My blog has proven to me that acupuncturists don't like this article, which means that I am successful at doing my job of stirring the pot of the healthcare world. Intramuscular stimulation, or IMS for short, is a fundamental part of my practice as a physiotherapist, but there are different regulations around the world as to whose scope of practice it falls into. It is a technique developed in Vancouver, Canada, by Dr. Chan Gunn. He worked with the Workers Compensation Board in the 1970s with countless injured workers and studied the roots of traditional Chinese acupuncture from a more Western-medicine approach, trying to apply our understanding of the neurophysiology of pain to explain why some acupuncture points seemed to work well for treating myofascial pain (pain experienced in the muscles and supporting connective tissue).

Before retiring, Dr. Gunn treated patients and collaborated with other doctors and a number of physical therapists in Vancouver at his non-profit center titled the Institute for the Study and Treatment of Pain (iSTOP). Together, they refined the use of acupuncture needles as a tool for treating chronic pain. The University of British Columbia sport medicine group has since taken over his mandate of research and training for the use of IMS by physiotherapists and physicians.

Acupuncturists argue that IMS simply is acupuncture, but as you can read in the comments section of my blog, I strongly disagree—as do thousands of clients who have experienced both forms of treatment. In Canada, IMS is primarily performed by physiotherapists, but the United States has a state-by-state bureaucratic battle underway to determine whether physical therapists are or are not allowed to perform the technique. A group called Kinetacore is trumpeting the cause for Americans, but, unfortunately, over-regulation has left the United States behind Canada and a handful of other countries in providing trained manual therapists, such as physiotherapists, the powerful tool that is IMS.

IMS is an anatomy-specific form of acupuncture performed by specially trained physiotherapists and some doctors. It is rooted in traditional Chinese acupuncture but is fundamentally different in many ways. IMS uses Western medicine's understanding of the neurophysiology of pain and Dr. Chan Gunn's assessment techniques of identifying underlying nerve irritations to treat chronic pain issues. The technique does use acupuncture needles, but not in the way someone practicing traditional acupuncture would. Traditional acupuncture focuses on pre-mapped-out points in the body that relate to different organs and meridians of energy. Fine acupuncture needles are then inserted into a number of these points and the person rests with them inserted for ten to twenty minutes. It can be very useful for the right condition, but it is not as specific or as purposeful as IMS for the treatment of pain.

When a physiotherapist performs IMS, they will first assess your basic posture and movement patterns to look for common signs of underlying nerve irritation. The most common one is to palpate (feel) for tender bands or knots in particular muscle groups.

They will look for restriction of movement in major joints such as your hips and shoulders and note the appearance of the skin and muscle tissue on either side of your spine. When there is an underlying nerve irritation in an area, the skin can start to look like the rind of an orange peel, feel thickened, and respond differently to light touch. A person may develop goose bumps easily and/or have areas of coolness or hair loss. The therapist will take all of these elements into account when determining where to treat you.

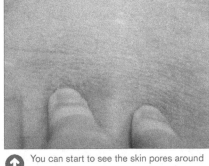

You can start to see the skin pores around the spine with the two-finger test when an underlying nerve is irritated.

IMS needles are slightly thicker than acupuncture needles, but would look exactly the same to the layperson. Once the physiotherapist has determined all the troubled areas, they will start using the needle to release them. The needle comes in a small plastic tube that is just slightly shorter than the needle. The plastic tube is pressed against the skin and the therapist quickly taps the end to push the fine needle through the skin. There is very minimal discomfort. The plastic tube is pulled off and the practitioner will push the end of the

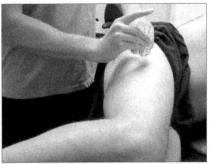

The tube is placed against skin, the end of needle tapped with finger.

needle further into the muscle. Here is a significant difference between IMS and acupuncture; in IMS, the needle is inserted deeper into the muscle and moved in and out to hunt and peck for bands of tight muscle tissue. The physiotherapist can feel the relative resistance to the movement of the needle and actively search for the stiffer, thicker-feeling areas; as the muscle releases, the relative resistance decreases. When inserting the needle, portions of the muscle can improve from feeling like a rubber eraser to a block of soft butter. The needle becomes an extension of the practitioner's hand to feel inside the muscle tissue.

If you put an acupuncture needle into a happy, healthy, normal muscle, little happens and the person doesn't feel much at all. On the other hand, if you put a needle into a muscle in a banded state, which is hypersensitive by nature, the stimulus will cause the muscle to contract and sometimes twitch. This contraction feels like a strong crampy ache, but it will only last five to ten seconds. Once the cramp is achieved, the needle is pulled back and the therapist moves on to the next point. The patient barely feels the needle; it is the muscle cramping that can be the uncomfortable part.

The physiotherapist will likely treat you in areas that you complained were hurting, but also in a variety of other parts that may not hurt but are part of the root cause of your problem. For example, most elbow problems are caused by an irritation of the C6 nerve root that extends out from the base of your neck; to fix your elbow, you would likely be needled around your neck, shoulder and arm first, then the forearm muscles if the elbow pain persists.

IMS, compared to acupuncture, is a more active process by the practitioner and requires a greater knowledge of anatomy, muscle balancing, and biomechanics to release the right areas and restore optimal movement. The ability to perform IMS provides the practitioner with a powerful tool to help eliminate chronic pain issues. It is the physiotherapist's ability, however, to assess and release tightness in the right order and to reintegrate proper movement patterns that make the real difference for the client. In other words, a client may find success with IMS with one practitioner and find it painful and not productive with another. There is an art and a science to it; the practitioner has been trained to use the science, but must develop the art with experience and the integration into rehabilitation and movement principle.

Many people either haven't heard about IMS or have been told that it is painful but works really well. What I tell people is that everyone's experience with IMS is different; some find it quite uncomfortable while others don't mind it at all. The difference seems to be related to both the person's body type and personality. People who are very muscular, tight, and compressed tend to find IMS the most painful, but still very effective. People with lower muscle tone are less bothered by the treatment. On the personality side, high-strung, type-A people experience trouble, because they are in a vulnerable position with involuntary muscle contraction, and find the lack of control stressful. That being said, they come back every time they hurt themselves asking for IMS, even though they hate every minute of it, because it works so well and they value the result over the temporary discomfort. I find people who are afraid of needles tend to do better with IMS than acupuncture, because they only have one needle in them at a time and only for ten seconds instead of ten minutes.

**So how does IMS work?**

Nerves are the electrical wiring to muscles. Muscles are a stringy, elastic tissue strung between two bones by tendons. In a normal resting state, the nerve supplies a steady signal to the muscle to create a normal resting tone so that it is not overly contracted or totally flaccid. When the nerve is irritated, it sends an altered signal to the muscle, making the muscle hyper-reactive; this usually results in bands of tension and muscle knots that are sore to the touch. These taut muscle bands don't allow the muscle to function properly, putting more stress on the tendons and joints when used. If you stick a fine needle into a muscle in its normal healthy state, not much happens and the client doesn't feel much, but if you stick a needle into a hypersensitive taut band the muscle will reflexively contract strongly or even twitch; this feels like a deep, crampy achy pressure to the client.

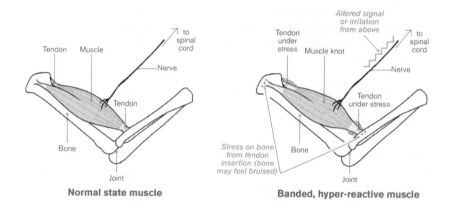

**Normal state muscle**                    **Banded, hyper-reactive muscle**

### Why make a tight, sore muscle contract more?

When the muscle contracts strongly, it stretches the tendons on either end that attach it to the bone. Your tendons have little stretch receptors embedded in them called Golgi tendon organs (GTO), and their job is to sense stretching and protect the muscle from contracting too strongly. When they are triggered, they reflexively send a signal to your spinal cord that immediately comes back saying, "relax, relax, relax" to the muscle. IMS effectively takes advantage of your body's own protective feedback loops and tricks your nervous system into dampening down the tone in specific muscle groups. People develop a love/hate relationship with it, because the crampy, achy feeling can be unpleasant, but it can produce immediate and lasting pain relief.

# Why Things Hurt: An IMS-Based Explanation

If you experience an acute accident or injury, like spraining your ankle, it is easy to understand why your ankle may hurt. You likely tore some of the ligaments and/or muscles around the joint and experienced subsequent swelling, bruising, and inflammation. Over a four-to-six-week period, your body typically fills in the torn tissue with scar tissue and slowly remodels it back to its original state. Sometimes, though, the pain persists beyond six weeks, even though the swelling and bruising have long since disappeared. Other times, pain appears for no apparent reason in the complete absence of an injury, and you can't understand why or what you did wrong.

Nerves are the electrical wiring of your body. They supply the energy for your muscles and organs to do their jobs. Your brain and spinal cord are like the electrical fuse box of your body, and your spine and skull are their protective coverings. Peripheral nerves extend from your spine at every level on both the left and right sides. The nerves that extend from your neck are responsible for most of the muscles in your shoulders, arms and hands, while the nerves that come from your lower back enervate all of the muscles in your hips, legs and feet. The nerves in the middle are responsible for your trunk and a lot of your organs.

Muscles are comprised of an abundance of stringy tissue that can stretch and contract. The muscle should possess a certain amount of resting tone; for example, at rest, it is slightly contracted and not flaccid or extremely tense—this is dictated by the input of the nerve. If the nerve is irritated as it extends from the spine, or anywhere in the periphery, it will result in an altered signal reaching the muscle. This altered signal can create bands of tension in the muscle, which will strain the joint and tendons, likely creating pain. Muscles are attached to bones on either side of a joint by tendons. Tendons are a tougher tissue that only stretch a small amount; when the muscle is in a banded state, the tendons endure a great deal more stress and strain when the joint is used, and the result is typically tendonitis.

To use your lower back as an example, let's look at your L3, 4 and 5 nerve roots as they extend from your spine. You will see that each nerve has its own hole to exit the spinal canal. The size of these holes is dependent on the level of

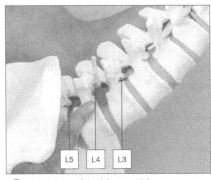

Locations of the L3, 4, and 5 nerve roots from the lower spine.

degeneration in your spine and discs, as well as the postures and movement strategies you use. Problems like disc herniations, bone spurs, and poor movement control lead to irritation of nerve roots as they extend from your spine. This will typically create bands of tension in the lower body and significantly lower the threshold of what it takes to injure or irritate muscles and nerves in the hips, legs and calves.

There are a number of common points of muscular tension that lead to chronic pain issues like sciatica and tennis elbow. The major nerve roots from your lower back turn into your sciatic nerve, which passes through the deep rotator muscles of your hip. Too much tension in these muscles can torsion your pelvis, compress your SI (sacroiliac) joint and irritate the nerve. The result may be pain and tension anywhere from your lower back, down the back of your leg to your calf and heel.

Similarly, the root cause of most chronic elbow pain stems from an irritation of your radial nerve due to tension in the back of the rotator cuff and compression in the base of the neck.

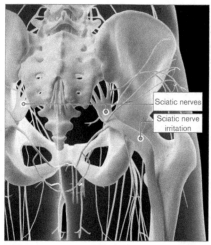

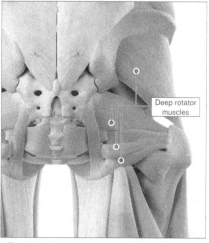

The major nerve roots from the lower back turn into the sciatic nerve.

The sciatic nerve passes through the deep rotator muscles of the hip.

Here is a simple illustration of a joint in a healthy, normal state. The muscle is resting in a gently contracted state with some elasticity between the two tendon attachments to the bones on either end. The nerve is supplying a steady signal from the spinal cord, and the joint should move freely and be pain free.

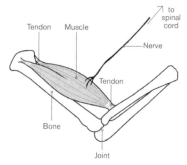

**Joint in normal, healthy state**

On the other hand, here we see an illustration of a joint in a painful state due to an underlying nerve irritation. Something has annoyed the nerve, which is causing it to send an altered signal to the muscle.

Imagine a flickering light bulb in a lamp when the wiring is off. The annoyed nerve causes the muscle to create bands of tension like muscle knots. The knots are typically tender to the touch, and the area may be colder due to poor blood flow through the tightened muscles. The increased tension in the muscle will compress the joint, ultimately leading to pain and potential degeneration over time. It can even make the bones feel bruised from the constant tug of the tendons.

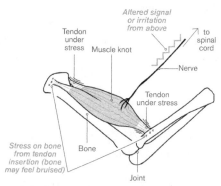

**Joint in painful state due to nerve irritation**

When nerves have been irritated for a long time, you will begin to notice subtle changes in the skin over the affected area, especially around the spine. Below is a picture of my father's back and neck, as a seventy-year-old lifetime athlete. He has a history of some back discomfort and was consistently pulling his calf muscles while playing tennis. You will notice as I run my two fingers up his spine, the skin and muscles in his lower back seem thickened and the pores start to look like the rind of an orange; this is a glaring sign of underlying nerve irritation, and the chronic calf strains he experienced were due to tension originating in the nerves in his lower back.

Pictured below (right) is the back of my father's neck. As you can see, he has a deep crease across the back, right around C5. This crease corresponded to significant degeneration in his neck at C4, 5 and 6 on a CT scan and resulted in enough nerve compromise to completely waste away some of his shoulder muscles. IMS

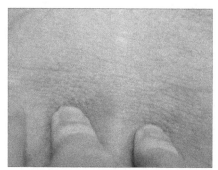

You can start to see the skin pores around the spine with the two-finger test when an underlying nerve is irritated.

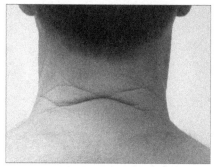

A deep crease across the back of the neck, right around C5, corresponded to a significant degeneration in the neck at C4, 5 and 6 as shown on a CT scan.

acupuncture kept him out of pain, but he ended up having surgery on his neck to clean up the degeneration and remove the strain on his nerve.

The muscle tension created by nerve irritations will typically make you feel as though you want to stretch out the muscle. Over-stretching muscles in this state, however, can actually make them tighten up even more. You are starting a tug-of-war with your body, and it is not a battle that you will win. When muscles are in a banded, irritated state, they will often act functionally weak, and the tendency of most therapists is to assign a person strengthening exercises to correct the problem. This can result in more pain by forcing the dysfunctional joint to do more work. The muscle is not typically weak; it is just not firing properly. It is important to release the tension before attempting even more exercise. IMS is a powerful tool to help unlock a muscle's potential and open a window for the person to re-educate the body to move properly again.

How you have learned to stand, sit, walk and breathe will affect the health and longevity of your spine and nervous system. IMS acupuncture is great at eliminating pain, but people are also great at creating it on their own. If you learn how to stand and move in a way that doesn't overly compress or hinge in your spine, you will experience far less pain throughout life.

# The Car Accident that Changed Everything: An IMS Success Story

Mindy came to me a broken person with no broken bones. She had been in a car accident a few years earlier that flipped her world upside down and sent her down a path of chronic pain, physical dysfunction, depression, and a diagnosis of complex regional pain syndrome (CRPS). In reflecting on our time together, I had no idea how low she was when I first met her. She was referred to me by an occupational therapist, named Lisa, who specialized in coordinating the rehabilitation of people who had been in accidents and needed some help navigating all their medical appointments. Usually, clients referred from Lisa had taken a few laps around the medical system, so I shouldn't have been surprised that Mindy was a complex case.

When we started, I was just another healthcare professional in a long, confusing maze where Mindy found herself; when we finished, I was the one who her daughter credited with saving her life. I realize now that she was completely numb to everything I said to her in our first appointment, because she had already seen specialist after specialist and her pain made anything I said just a collection of meaningless words. I assessed her and spent a significant amount of time explaining what I believed to be the problem. Then, with her consent, I performed IMS on her hips and lower back. I didn't see her again for two months.

Mindy had been a banker before her accident. She was married, with two kids in their early twenties, and had lived a moderately active lifestyle. The intense, jarring forces of her car accident left her with acute sprains and strains in her body, but no vital injuries. She went through the typical course of anti-inflammatories, physiotherapy, and check-ups with her family doctor before attempting a gradual return to work a month or two later. She was a motivated woman who attempted to return to her normal life even though she was still in pain. Unfortunately, her return to work didn't last long, because she was just too uncomfortable to concentrate on her job, so she took more time off and went back to physiotherapy and prescription painkillers.

Mindy was experiencing pain in her back, neck, arms, and legs, and found that her mobility for day-to-day tasks seemed to be getting worse. Her family doctor cycled her through a variety of different medications before referring her to a physiatrist. She had to wait four months to see the specialist, during which time Mindy was off work and fighting with her insurer to cover the costs of her physical therapy and massage treatments. She tried a few different therapists in that time, but her symptoms continued to worsen; she was holding on to hope that the specialist would provide some answers after the long wait.

The physiatrist spent an hour with Mindy, talking through her history, and examining her. In the end, he came to the conclusion that she was suffering from "soft tissue injuries" as a result of her car accident, and that she should be enrolled in an occupational rehabilitation program that consisted of group exercise and education sessions four hours a day, five days per week, supervised by a physiotherapist and a kinesiologist. He wrote a report for her doctor and otherwise offered little help. She was frustrated and disappointed that, after a four-month wait, the only thing that the specialist could do for her was recommend more exercise.

Based on the doctor's recommendations, Mindy ended her one-on-one physiotherapy coverage, and she started the remedial group version of what she was already doing without success. Mindy's legs started swelling, her skin turned shiny, and walking became more and more difficult, until she had to stop the group program and stay at home in pain. At that point, her insurer wanted her to see one of their specialists, her lawyer wanted her to see one of his specialists, and her family doctor referred her to a pain clinic that had over a year-long waiting list. I entered into her life in the middle of this period when her pain was getting worse and her perspective seemed less and less hopeful. She hadn't worked in a few years, walking was a chore, and she stayed at home depressed most of the time.

Mindy was too depressed to follow my explanations, and my first IMS session only made her sore, so she retreated for a few months until Lisa convinced her to give me another try. With a new respect for her situation, I altered my approach and had her buy into understanding how IMS might help her. Months into our treatment, she visited a neurologist who confirmed a diagnosis of CRPS, a chronic pain condition caused by malfunction of the nervous system, resulting in painfully swollen limbs. Mindy's lower legs and feet were swollen and hypersensitive to the world around them. Her hips were locked up and her arms felt swollen and sore but didn't look as bad as her legs. I could tell that she felt like her body was no longer her own. She moved with a lethargy and lack of control that was biomechanically making her pain much worse.

When you lift one foot off the ground, the other foot, ankle, knee, hip, and sacroiliac (SI) joint transfer the load to your pelvis and trunk to keep you standing properly; the combination of pain and tension in Mindy's lower body completely disrupted how she was supposed to move, leaving her with more pain and no idea about how to return to normal. It was my job to get her to a place where she could help herself again, because she had nearly given up when we started. I began by performing IMS to the deep rotator muscles of both her hips and the deep spinal stabilizing muscles of her lower back. Although her pain did not dramatically change, her functional mobility improved significantly after four sessions over a month's time.

I could start to see that Mindy's hips and pelvis were working together with the muscles in her legs to stabilize her properly, allowing her to balance and move around more comfortably. Her overall well-being seemed to improve, because she could get out for walks again and not feel quite so helpless. She started to see a flicker of hope that her body was turning around, instead of sinking deeper down the tunnel of dysfunction. I progressed to doing IMS up her entire spine to her neck, her shoulder muscles and down to her calves. They were long and uncomfortable sessions for Mindy, but she saw it as a necessary evil, because it was giving her a life back. She slowly began activities like yoga and gardening for her physical and mental well-being. It was a big step for her to be doing things that she enjoyed again, because depression, along with the stress of the looming lawsuit with her auto insurance company, had taken a hold of her and became entangled with her pain.

Over a period of months, I saw Mindy's function improve significantly, and over the year I saw the skin changes in her legs start to revert to a more normal appearance; it was her pain and the impact the journey had on her as a person that was hard to gauge. I saw her go through the series of medical specialist frustrations, the legal discovery process with the lawyers, and the result of getting a large financial settlement a few years later. Although she was satisfied with her settlement and relieved to be done with the legal proceedings, her depression took a turn for the worse because now she was left with no job or direction for the future, and she was still living with pain as part of her new identity.

We progressed Mindy to a maintenance stage of doing IMS about once per month to calm her nervous system and to help her with her pain. It was then when I started my own journey of injury, pain, perseverance and a new sense of empathy.

I took three months off of work after a serious eye injury, lying around in bed and stuck at home in pain, which was ample time for me to start feeling down about my situation and reflect on some of the paths I have seen clients follow after life-changing injuries. It was difficult to avoid depression and to look at life objectively when everything seemed to be going wrong. I had low moments, days, and even weeks, but it was my experience of helping people through their own journeys that gave me the mental framework needed to get back to work and take control of my life as soon as I could, even though I was still in pain and had horrible double vision.

I saw Mindy again a few months after I returned from my time off. She was continuing with yoga, started photography lessons, and did a regular aquafit class to keep her busy and moving. She still reported daily pain and seemed lost in the world, but was thriving compared to where she was a year earlier, and needed time to shed pain as an identity. IMS was the life preserver that pulled her out of the darkness, but her next step was to take back control so that she could really enjoy life again. I have helped her and learned from her, and I am still trying to support her recovery which may be a few more years in the making.

We all need people in our lives to support us and give us perspective, both looking forward and looking back. Bad things happen to good people all the time, and the best thing you can help them do—when they are ready—is to accept that it happened and to build a framework in moving forward within their new "normal." Perspective is the most important aspect to gain, but it is more difficult to develop when you are zoomed into the moment-to-moment suffering of pain and dysfunction. It is the job of friends, family, and healthcare workers to provide the support, direction, and objectivity necessary to help a person lost in chronic pain to pan out and look at their life as a journey. I have to work on keeping this perspective every day, and hopefully Mindy too will get there soon.

# How Your Organs May Be the Problem: Understanding Visceral and Neural Manipulation

Visceral manipulation is the practice of an experienced therapist using his hands to move and release fascial restrictions in your abdomen and pelvis to encourage the normal movement and function of your internal organs. Most people are familiar with the idea of joint and muscle restrictions causing tightness, pain, and limited movement in their bodies but don't consider the role of their organs. It is common for people to visit their physiotherapist, chiropractor, or massage therapist to treat pain and alignment issues; unfortunately, if they are not considering the mobility of your organs in your alignment and movement patterns, these practitioners may only be treating the outer shell of the problem.

As of this writing, I have been a physiotherapist for thirteen years and have continued to add layers of knowledge and skills to my tool belt. Two of those skills have been real eye openers and game-changers for me. The first was the profound effectiveness of skilled dry needling called IMS. The second was a series of osteopathic manual therapy techniques called visceral and neural manipulation. I had previously been taught how every joint in the body works, where all the muscles attach and which nerves innervate them, but I had not been educated on how the inside of the body affects the outside. The combination of training in IMS and visceral work gave me the ability to effectively treat the body as a whole.

Visceral and neural manipulation have helped me to understand just how connected everything really is. Neural manual therapy allows me to assess and treat the nervous system by gently manipulating the membranes and nerves in the head, face and limbs to help the body make sense of its own interconnectedness. I was cynical to start but have been blown away by how powerful a tool this specific and purposeful light touch can be.

The bones of your skull, face and mouth are much more movable than one would think, and they greatly impact your nervous system as a whole. Car accidents, blows to the face, and dental work all have the capacity to create torsioning forces in your head, which can have a rippling effect throughout your body. I fixed one lady's chronic left leg pain by releasing tension from the joint where her face meets her head. I dramatically changed another man's whiplash-related neck and shoulder pain by treating a membrane in his brain called the tentorium through his temporal bones, just behind his ears. Neural manipulation has given me the ability to treat the connections of the head to the body, the head to the organs, and the head to the limbs in a way I didn't realize was possible.

Your trunk and pelvis form a bony, muscular, fascial outer shell to protect and encase all of your internal organs. Your organs are not loosely floating around in there, though; they are mostly supported by tissue called fascia and pleura. The organs are in a sealed system under pressure that squishes everything tightly together; each organ is wrapped in its own pleura and bathed in fluid so it can slide around its neighboring organs. Issues that affect the pressures in the system or the ability of the organs to move around in their close quarters will affect the ability of the body to move and function properly.

Pregnancy, abdominal surgery, infection, jarring injuries, and emotional behaviors can all affect the mobility of your organs or viscera. Pregnancy involves a great deal of stretching and reorganizing of almost everything in a woman's abdomen; this happens gradually over nine months, and the body, amazingly, figures out how to create space for a whole other person in there. The issues can arise more so during and after labor when everything is asked to change in a relatively short period of time. There is a significant pressure change, and all of a sudden organs can start dropping back down; whether they find their proper, functional place depends on how the labor went, how much damage occurred to the supportive muscles, and whether surgery was performed.

The C-section is a much more invasive surgery than most people realize, but any abdominal surgery will create "stickiness" in the viscera. As I mentioned, your organs are bathed in a small amount of fluid to allow them to slide around as you move; any time you expose the abdomen to air and surgical lights, dryness or stickiness is bound to occur, which restricts the normal mobility of the organs. A therapist trained in visceral manipulation by means of light touch can assess and treat any restrictions to help restore mobility.

Because the fascial wrappings of your organs are essentially one long, continuous piece of connective tissue, restrictions in one area can manifest as symptoms in other areas. A good analogy is to wear a relatively tight T-shirt and twist a piece in one corner into a knot. You will likely see and feel the pull from your lower-left abdomen all the way up in your right shoulder; this same concept effectively happens inside you. Your body will start to "hug" or protect the area of restriction, which leads to alignment issues and compensatory movement

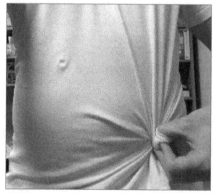

It helps to understand how the fascial wrappings of your organs work with a T-shirt knot-twist, simulating the same pull that can happen inside you.

patterns. Alignment problems and poor movement patterns often lead to pain and tension in the bony and muscular systems; treating these usually helps provide relief, but if the problem returns, it is likely that the root of the problem may be a visceral restriction.

Though relatively new to using visceral manipulation as a treatment modality, I have already found it to be the missing puzzle piece for many of my clients who have stubborn, persistent pain issues. It is an entirely painless, light-touch form of manual therapy that requires therapists to know their anatomy extensively. Used in conjunction with other forms of manual therapy, dry needling, and movement training, it makes most conditions treatable by conservative means.

Jarring forces involved in sports, car accidents, and falls can affect your organs just as much as your muscles and bones. The shear forces can create tearing and scar tissue, and the impact can create bruising. Your body does its best to protect vital organs during extreme forces, but in doing so can create an aftermath of restrictions that may result in pain. Therapists should consider that the driving issue behind their client's pain could be coming from something inside which may be harder to reach than simply treating the muscles.

The emotional piece was one of the most interesting aspects about visceral work. To paraphrase the late osteopath Dr. John Upledger, our organs echo our emotions. You may have a "gut feeling" or "butterflies in your stomach." In stressful or intense situations, your brain passes the stress onto your organs and creates an organ-behavior relationship. Each person tends to have his or her own weak link in a particular organ, and this relates to their underlying personality traits.

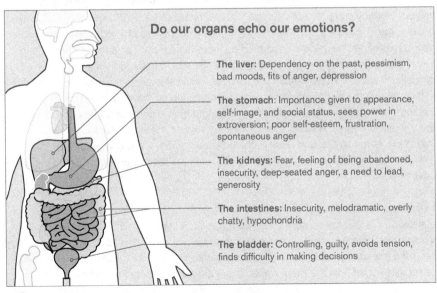

### Do our organs echo our emotions?

**The liver:** Dependency on the past, pessimism, bad moods, fits of anger, depression

**The stomach:** Importance given to appearance, self-image, and social status, sees power in extroversion; poor self-esteem, frustration, spontaneous anger

**The kidneys:** Fear, feeling of being abandoned, insecurity, deep-seated anger, a need to lead, generosity

**The intestines:** Insecurity, melodramatic, overly chatty, hypochondria

**The bladder:** Controlling, guilty, avoids tension, finds difficulty in making decisions

A few examples taken from Upledger's poster, "Understanding Your Organs."

These are only a few examples, but the concept makes sense to me as a physiotherapist. I see people all the time who seem to have a back or a shoulder that always "goes out" on them at the most inopportune times. They have no idea what they did and don't understand why it comes back two or three times a year. They have done all the core classes they could find, but strength just wasn't the issue. Their chronic issue is where their body holds stress and how it protectively reacts around it. Stress is a powerful force, and your organs are the crossover between physical and mental well-being.

The fascinating part of the osteopathic approach to treating pain is that it can provide explanations based purely on anatomy for very common but poorly understood ailments. Frozen shoulder can relate to a nerve irritation stemming from the visceral pleura. Chronically cold feet can be your small intestines. Persistent left sciatica or sacroiliac (SI) pain can be your sigmoid colon. Right medial knee pain and instability can be an irritation of your obturator nerve near your large intestine. Right shoulder pain can be a restriction in your liver. Heartburn and gastric reflux can mean your stomach is sitting too high. It is more complicated than I make it sound, but the amazing part is that it is all treatable by a good manual therapist who knows his anatomy inside and out (literally).

Visceral manipulation is unlikely to be the answer for everything, but it could be the solution for a lot of people. If you want to find a practitioner who uses visceral manipulation, you are best to start looking in this order: an osteopath, a registered massage therapist, a physiotherapist, or a naturopath.

Your brain is separated in two halves by a membrane down the center called the falx, and each half is supported by a similar membrane on each side called the tentorium. These membranes absorb forces that your body goes through during normal movement and during jarring forces to help protect your nervous system from being damaged or injured, but they can hold onto tension that can affect your cranial alignment and tension down a whole side of your body. People regularly come in to physiotherapy a few years after a rear-ender car accident complaining that the whole left side of their body doesn't seem to like them; their hip is locked up, their shoulder hurts and their ankle doesn't move like it should. These people usually have a cranial torsion stemming from tension in their tentorium paired with a fascial organ restriction on the same side. Previously, I simply used IMS to help straighten them out, but have since found that addressing the deeper driving force behind the asymmetry with neural manipulation has translated into much longer lasting and more profound improvements. The combination of skilled manual therapy and precise dry needling can really reintegrate the two sides of the body back together.

Learning neural manipulation has been the framework that helped make visceral manipulation make sense to me; the two forms of treatment dovetail together perfectly. Visceral and neural manipulation are skills that require years to master, but the process can be a rewarding one that will help a healthcare practitioner develop a deeper understanding of how the body works. There are therapists and courses around the world that utilize and teach these skills, and I believe it is simply a matter of time before the practice becomes more mainstream.

# The Lady Who Slept and Showered in Her Shoes: The Role of Stress, Anxiety, and Fear on Pain

Beatrice was referred to me by a local pain specialist for her chronic bilateral foot pain. She was a very pleasant lady in her early sixties who loved singing almost as much as she loved her infant grandson. She alternated days singing in a choir and caring for the baby, but her feet caused her endless problems no matter which pastime she was doing. By the time she found herself in my office, Beatrice had four pairs of the exact same orthopedic-looking running shoes—two pairs in white and two pairs in black—with custom-built orthotics in all of them, and she was afraid to take them off. She slept in her shoes to protect her feet and sat on a chair in the shower with shoes on to prevent them from hurting. Then she met me.

I am not a fan of orthotics (refer to Section 4, "Shoes: Good Support or Coffins for Your Feet?") but she didn't know that at the time. She was focused on her feet, and as far as she knew, everything she was doing was the best-available option, so she did it religiously. She had bed shoes, shower shoes, inside shoes and outside shoes—a variety of coffins that ensured her painful feet would never see the light of day. Her doctor had prescribed high doses of a nerve drug, which she felt was making a big difference, so she also became fixated and ceremonious about her pills. I learned very quickly that Beatrice was an extremely particular person, driven by anxiety and fear: anxiety that she had to do everything just perfectly to contain the fear of making her pain worse.

Beatrice had rigid, high-arched feet with some arthritic change and tension in her calves. She walked looking at the floor two inches in front of her, in short staccato strides that didn't require her ankle to move very much. She only went out for rehearsal or babysitting duties; otherwise her foot pain was largely keeping her inside the house. Her life was being held hostage by her feet and how she was dealing with them, so I started my mission to free Beatrice's feet from her mind. While she absolutely had physical issues responsible for her discomfort, I needed to chisel away at her mindset if I was going to get anywhere.

Anxious people become very controlling of their environment to help sooth their minds, so I knew that I wasn't going change Beatrice's mind on anything cold turkey. I had to earn her trust and be careful to not push her too far outside of her tightly monitored boundaries. I started by using IMS to loosen her calves and tried to draw her attention to how she was walking. She looked ridiculous and needed someone to call her on it.

All that I asked her to change was to look forward instead of down and to take slower, longer strides. She laughed at my imitation of her walk and didn't find my task too scary, so we had a starting point.

Beatrice's gait pattern was going to take some time to change, so the next behavior that I targeted was her practice of sleeping in her shoes and orthotics. I explained that her orthotics would only do some possible good if she was standing on them, so I encouraged her to, at very least, remove her orthotics while sleeping to give her feet a bit more room to move in her shoes. My appeal to reason seemed to work, and my first victory was her sleeping in just her shoes after three weeks of seeing me. I saw her once a week regularly for months, where I would perform IMS on her hips, back, calves, and feet while systematically trying to extract her from her shoes. Beatrice found the IMS treatment really loosened her up, and she quickly ritualized it as one of the treatments that she required to function. I was okay with her depending on the needles, because it was my way in to modifying her behavior.

We spent time walking around my treatment room with her in bare feet, a practice that she never did at home. I slowly convinced her to take the orthotics out of her orthopedic shoes and replace them with a simple metatarsal pad. I challenged her need to wear shoes to bed every single time she came in; I wasn't pushy, but I was consistent and eventually she went to bed without them—a huge victory for both of us. She progressively started feeling more confident about her feet and, very slowly, started weaning off her nerve medication. Again, I didn't push her on it; I just consistently suggested she try less drugs. We peeled away her security blankets and found that her pain didn't get better or worse. So we kept peeling.

The next task was to stop her need for shower shoes. In my mind, if Beatrice could walk around my office in bare feet, she could have a shower without having to get her shoes all wet, but I couldn't flat out say that. We continued to loosen her up with IMS and I continued to challenge her current assumptions, and over a few months we had her sleeping in super-thick socks and showering while standing on face cloths, two major improvements for her day-to-day life. Beatrice seemed quite positive throughout the entire process. She was resistant to change all the way along, but was proud of her accomplishments and firm in her boundaries. She didn't outwardly project fear and anxiety about her pain, but her behavior screamed it, even as she worked to conquer it.

Once I had firmly gained her trust, I started trying visceral and neural manipulation work to see if I could provide her with more physical relief. I found her small intestines to be a ball of tension, as well as a mild cranial torsion that seemed to be contributing to her foot and calf tension on her right side. If anything, it was a good distraction from her perceived need for the IMS and something that could distract her attention from her feet. I worked hard to try and provide her relief from her physical symptoms, but I made further gains in her cognitive ones. I convinced her to buy a pair of New Balance Minimus Zero shoes to wear around her house, a compromise I was happy with if I couldn't get her to go barefoot, and a huge improvement from the clunky shoes with orthotics that she was living in before.

Beatrice started to replace her need for overly supportive shoes with her need to see me on a regular basis. After a number of months, though, I forced a break in our treatment pattern when I went on vacation for three weeks. From what I could tell when I returned, her functional pain level was much the same, but her behavior had regressed in my absence. Three weeks without me resulted in her giving up her minimalist shoes and stopping her slow wean of medication, and it took me another full month to get her back to our previous accomplishments. I knew Beatrice was going to require a long-term strategy that involved me, at most, once per month without her backtracking, but I wasn't sure how to begin this process. I allowed myself to be her new security blanket while she enjoyed a more normal home life for a few months and then gradually tried to convince her to visit less and less.

It took over a year to progress Beatrice to a reasonable maintenance plan, but we did it and I am very proud of her. I learned a great deal about patience and individual needs in working with her. She came to me looking for help with her pain, but I can't say that I took it away for her; I just helped her to deal with it in a more functional manner. She showed me how powerfully the brain can amplify the perception of pain and how consuming it can become in one's life. She also taught me that patience, persistence, and non-judgmental help can change even the deepest-rooted behaviors. I still see Beatrice today and enjoy the chess match of mental suggestion that slowly pushes her toward a more normal and pain-free life.

# Mindfulness: The Skill of Living in the Present

Mindfulness is a concept that was introduced to me in my mid-twenties while I was working at Diane Lee's physiotherapy clinic in South Surrey, British Columbia, with a caseload comprised largely of chronic pain clients and seniors. I was at a stage where I was still able to be selfish with my personal time and hadn't gained the perspective that marriage, kids, a mortgage, and personal injury later provided me. I learned concepts from Daniel Siegel's book Mindsight that I thought would help me work with my clients more effectively, which they did, but they more so prepared me for the transition to real adult life that exploded into reality in my thirties.

Experience creates wisdom, if you are aware of what is happening to you in the present and are able to reflect on it in a meaningful way later in life; but experience without this awareness can create confusion, fear, and anxiety. The latter, unfortunately, is what happens to many people who suffer from accidents, injuries, and pain; they have a negative physical experience and have very little context with which to understand what is happening to their bodies. It is almost impossible to step back and look at your situation objectively unless you understand the principles of how your body and your brain process trauma. The two are intimately connected, and what Dr. Siegel calls "mindsight:" the concept of tapping into the dance that's happening in your head which creates the lens through which you see the world. It is a powerful skill to acknowledge your own biases and filters with the ability to explain your own behaviors through basic scientific principle.

Thankfully, I learned the concept of mindfulness from a book before I really needed it. The principles made sense to me and helped me better understand some of my clients, my family, and my friends. In hindsight, I first took everything I learned about the topic and applied it to my understanding of other people before I really absorbed that I needed to apply it to myself. It's much easier to analyze other people than to delve into your own inner workings, but I feel that whatever opens the door to self-awareness is a good first step. Some people—myself included—require a significant event or experience to shift their perspective from outward to inward. I am thankful that I had laid the mental groundwork of self-awareness before I had three kids in three years, started a business, and then suffered a serious injury. I associate the mindfulness I have developed in the past ten years with my success as a father, a husband, an entrepreneur, and a patient.

Google Maps is a good analogy for looking at your life, in your ability to zoom right into your rooftop from a satellite in space, or all the way out to your continent, or anything in between. The skill of doing this with your own life is a powerful tool that a person can develop for their own mental health. Some people spend far too much time zoomed right into their own rooftop and lose perspective of what their neighbors are thinking and doing, while others zoom way out until they are lost looking at a map of North America and can't figure out where they fit in. Spending too much time on either end of the spectrum can make a person forget that life is lived in the middle zone and that you need to be able to switch between different views in order to not take yourself too seriously, to love yourself, to love others, and to create direction in your life. Different life events tend to make people park in one view too long and then have trouble navigating the different aspects of their lives that require multiple perspectives.

Becoming a parent, I believe, is the biggest paradigm shift a person can undergo and the biggest controller of the zoom button. Witnessing my own little human come into the world after an intense thirty-six-hour labor was a surreal experience and an emotional roller coaster for both my wife and me. My job was to support her through the most physically draining and uncomfortable experience humans naturally endure. It was a helpless place for me, watching her hit the wall a few times, but I tried my best to keep her going through her four hours of pushing, which eventually ended when the obstetrician swooped in and took over from the midwife and pulled my son out. He was having trouble breathing and I was given a mini oxygen mask to hold over his little mouth.

I had spent the previous day and a half so intensely focused on my wife, when all of a sudden I seemed to be on the medical team for this new little person and was told to follow them as we left my exhausted wife behind. I watched as nurses hooked my little guy up to monitoring lines and placed him in a closed incubator in a room with ten other struggling babies. I'm not sure how long I stayed there before I asked if I could go back and see my wife, but it felt like an eternity. I have never had the outside world disappear more from my conscious awareness than that forty-eight-hour period.

My son was eventually fine, but his traumatic entrance to this world left a significant impact on our family. My wife and son stayed in the hospital for longer than usual, and my role in the situation was like a monkey took over the zoom button. I went from the intensity of the hospital to the outside world, to our eerily empty house, to having to start thinking about work again and back to the hospital—on repeat in every imaginable order. I was self-employed in my relatively new business, so there was no paid vacation time. Finances hung over my head, and I started learning how to balance the real world that was still happening with my wife who was zoomed right in to the ordeals of caring for a high-maintenance new baby.

Over the following year, my wife had the challenge of staying so zoomed in to one aspect all the time, while I had to develop the art of seamlessly changing gears from baby, to work, to happy wife, to finances, to sleep, to sad wife, to poo, to pee, to frustrated wife and back to work, in an order that was constantly shifting. It was an exercise in perspective that built my character, changed my values and taught me what love really is. Three times in three years was a bit aggressive, but eight years later I have to agree with the saying, "What doesn't kill you makes you stronger."

I have learned how much a person's perspective affects their attitude about life by getting the opportunity to dive deep into parenting, but also being forced to step away from it for eight to ten hours a day, five days a week, while my wife eats, sleeps and breathes it twenty-four hours a day. I get the chance to develop objectivity about our family life by stepping back from it while she is the locomotive that keeps it all going. I miss out on a lot of fun moments throughout the day, but am able to enjoy the ones I do have more, because I haven't been worn down by the daily grind of a four-, five- and seven-year-old's needs. When we come together to parent, I have to be able to appreciate hers and my filter, because our days are typically different up to that point and it can be easy to butt heads. My mindfulness has been a skill that I've relied on to help get my family through a chaotic seven years, and it is a tool that I try my best to keep developing.

In September 2011, my worlds collided to challenge what I thought I was just getting the hang of. We had our third child in three years, we moved and expanded our physiotherapy clinic, and my business partner was hospitalized with an unknown illness for a month—oh, and my receptionist quit—all at the same time. I had an infant, an eighteen-month-old, a three-year-old, and a new clinic that needed to be launched while trying to treat my clients without a receptionist! I'm sure I learned something from that process, but it was all a blur. I made it through, jumping back and forth between all my duties, and eventually came up for air a few years later.

Perseverance and hard work have given me three healthy kids, a loving wife, and a thriving business. It started as just me and a cheap massage table from Costco in a private room of a fitness center, and now I have two private clinics with seven physiotherapists, three massage therapists, three kinesiologists, and four Pilates instructors. When life challenges you, you just have to keep moving forward, in as big or small an increment as you can muster, and you will eventually end up where you want to be. Awareness of your own capacity at any given time is the key to not burning out.

In August of 2014, my busy life came screeching to a halt when I was struck in the right eye by an orange floor hockey ball. Business was going well, the kids were becoming easier to handle and life was good, and then one day it all stopped. My zoom button became focused right in on me. I was thrown into a downward spiral of surgeries and procedures that left me bedridden for three months with pain, nausea, and all-round badness. I went from having every minute of every day filled with something to do, to being stuck in bed in my mother's condo having trouble even being vertical, thinking straight, or eating anything. Doing nothing all of a sudden became harder than doing everything all at once, and the outside world seemed more and more distant as the surgeries, medications, and my vision got progressively worse with time.

My wife and kids tried to visit me, but I didn't have anything to offer to the people who were technically my dependents. I had to focus on myself to get through the ordeal and come out the other side as a loving father and husband. I battled with depression after four surgeries in three months and pushed myself to get back to work to create some normalcy in my life. I returned to a shell-shocked family and a caseload of clients who couldn't help but talk about what happened to me, because my eye was visibly painful and awkwardly crooked. Through the following year, I worked at mending fences at home, treating my clients, and endured three more surgeries that didn't help my vision; it was an exercise in resilience that I will never forget and am still working through.

Stoicism requires objectivity and rational thought, which are two things that can be almost impossible to achieve when you find yourself in a really difficult situation, but that is when they are needed most. It is okay to be sad, angry, and frustrated about your place in life, but it is your ability to accept that the bad things happened to you, make it your own, and to look at your future with purpose that will prevent depression from sinking its teeth into you. It took me the better part of a year to regain enough confidence in myself after being so badly rattled by what I went through. Although I can't say that I am better off for having gone through it, I have gained a new level of awareness for the role of mental health in individuals and society.

Make sure that you check in with yourself on a regular basis and question how you feel, what you are doing, and where you are going, because knowing yourself will make you all the more resilient should adversity strike. No matter how many responsibilities you have in life, the best way you can help others is to take care of yourself, mentally and physically. Other people will do crazy, annoying, and dangerous things around you, and your best defense is to own your space, own your thoughts, and own your reactions—a practice that is accomplished by the process of mental and physical awareness, or mindfulness.

# My Eye Injury: A Physical and Emotional Battle

This section contains three separate posts that I cathartically wrote on my blog after my eye injury. The first one was written after I first returned to work; the second was around the one-year anniversary of my accident; and the third was one month after my seventh and final surgery, nineteen months later.

**Return to Work Three Months after Accident:**
**Written November 26, 2014**

This story is a detailed account of how I spent the fall of 2014. A big part of me wants to forget everything that happened over those three months, but something inside of me wants to tell the story. I warn you: every time I go into detail about what I went through, people squirm and shy away. It was the darkest, lowest part of my life to date, and I am only beginning to re-establish some normalcy for my family and business. I returned to work just a few weeks ago, three weeks following my fourth eye surgery in two months after I was struck in the right eye with a hard orange floor hockey ball on August 19, 2014.

My wife and three children were away at our family cabin. I had returned to work for the week after an amazing almost three-week holiday, but I only made it to Tuesday before my world changed. Earlier in the summer, a client had told me about a regular pick-up floor hockey game at a nearby community center. I played a few times before my vacation, but I was the new guy among a group that had been playing together for a while. The only guy that I somewhat knew was my client.

The game was social, but competitive. Every guy had a different level of protective gear, but most did not have any form of eye protection. I happened to have my squash goggles with me, but I was running late and forgot them in the car. I had never worn eye protection while playing floor hockey before but was definitely considering it with this group; unfortunately, I never got the chance. I decided to jump right into the game and was having a great time. I scored five goals in the first two games before it happened. I ended up in the corner just off to the side of net. I turned back to follow the ball when I saw, for a split second, an orange ball flying right at my face.

I have managed to hurt most parts of my body over the years, and the immediate question in my mind is: "Are you hurt or are you injured?" This time it took a full ten seconds to realize that I was in trouble. I dropped to my knees in pain, and a slow trickle of blood dripped from my nose. My eyeball hurt, and my vision was 100% gone in that eye. One of the guys on the floor was a doctor. He covered my eye with a patch and helped me call my father to take me to the hospital. It turns out the guy who shot the ball was my client. He felt awful, but all he was guilty of was a bad shot.

Sitting at the Vancouver General Hospital (VGH) emergency room that night, I had no idea how intense of a physical and emotional journey I was about to begin. Trips to the ER were not foreign to me, but this injury took me well beyond the ER. I was triaged into the "eye room" that seemed to be full of equipment that the ER doctors only somewhat knew how to use, and had done so very occasionally. A few doctors fumbled around with tools to measure the pressure in my eye, unsuccessfully, before they said that I was in luck and the ophthalmology resident was close by. He would see me at the eye care center down the street. The doctor highlighted the building on a map and said goodbye and good luck. By this time it was 10:30 p.m., and I was walking by myself in the dark with one eye looking for a specific building. As I advanced to the right block, I heard a man call out, "Floor hockey?" It was the ophthalmology resident standing outside the building. It was closed, but he opened it up to bring me and one other man into the clinic.

The other man seemed to have spilled a chemical in his eye, but it sounded like he was going to be fine and the resident sent him home relatively quickly. Then he turned his attention to me and spent nearly an hour looking at my eye with every tool he had, all the while making little comments about this being quite a bad injury. I began to realize that my lack of vision might not be temporary. He finally told me to meet him back here the next morning at 9 a.m. and he would get me in to see the retinal specialist. I was sent home with a patch on my eye and a prescription for some eye drops.

My dad drove me home that night with a pit stop at Shoppers Drug Mart on Broadway to pick up my prescription. He left me in the car on a hot August night while he ran in to fill my prescription. After about five minutes, I felt extremely nauseous and threw up all over the sidewalk of one of the busiest streets in Vancouver. It was beginning.

I slept okay that night, all things considered; my eye hurt, but the vomiting seemed under control. I returned to the eye care center the next morning, but this time it was full with hundreds and hundreds of people between the ages of sixty and eighty-five. There was barely anywhere to sit, and the air conditioning was on full blast. My dad dropped me off in shorts, a T-shirt and flip-flops to a meat locker full of old people who all looked as though they had been sitting there for two hours already, and it was only 9 a.m. I checked in and was taken right away to see the doctor from the night before. He ordered a retinal scan and an angiogram immediately, and then promptly walked me over to Dr. Ma's office, a very busy retinal specialist who had treated National Hockey League centerman Manny Malhotra's eye injury. I was happy to be seen so quickly, but understood that being triaged to the top of the list was likely not a good thing!

Dr. Ma looked at my eye and the test results and informed me that I was going to need surgery to try and remove the blood from behind my retina. He sent me back out to the waiting room where a nurse helped me fill out the paperwork for my surgery. I understood the back of my eye was damaged and that Dr. Ma was going to try and fix it. I was told to rest for two days until my surgery. At this point, I had zero vision in my right eye; it was just darkness. I developed a nice black eye and had a headache. Looking back, though, I didn't feel so bad, all things considered.

Then I had surgery. Most eye surgeries are done under local anesthetic, where you are sedated but conscious for the procedure. It didn't sound like a great idea to me, but I trusted them in that it wouldn't hurt. Guess what? It hurt! They performed what is called a vitrectomy with the insertion of a gas bubble into my eye, which means they suck out the vitreous fluid from my eye and replace it with a gas bubble. I then lay face down for the next three to five days in attempt to have the gas bubble press into the hemorrhage on the back of my eye and hopefully push out the blood from behind my retina. Apparently, I also had an orbital floor fracture (the bottom of the eye socket), which is why the tugging and pulling of the procedure hurt. The freezing they gave me didn't affect this bone. Lucky me.

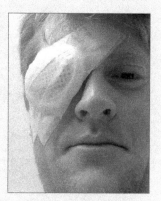

In the recovery room, the nurses had me flip onto my stomach and told me I would have to stay in this position 90% of the time for the next three to five days. I was free to go home once my pain level was below a four out of ten. It took two Tylenol 3s, Gravol and two oxycodone to push me below a four and be sent home. My wife and three young children were still at our cabin, so my mother and father-in-law were my nurses and taxi drivers. I don't know what I would have done without them. My mother rented a set of cushions designed for lying face down, and my business partner Harry borrowed a colleague's portable massage table for my face-down sentence.

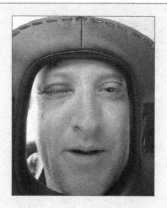

I had a pretty good attitude at first. I had an injury. I had a surgery to fix it. I figured three days face down wasn't the end of the world if it would save my vision. The first forty-eight hours were uncomfortable, but I managed. Beyond that point, however, I started to sense that something was wrong. I just couldn't stay face down, because my eye was hurting and my face couldn't tolerate the pressure of being rested upon. I started taking the Tylenol 3s, but they only left me feeling awful and didn't help the pain. I shifted to my side and tried to stay looking down. I kept thinking in the back of my head, *you need to stay face down or you might not get your vision back.* I held out longer than I probably should have, but by two o'clock in the morning I woke up my mom and told her I wasn't doing well.

My mom tried paging the resident ophthalmologist on-call, but technology in a sleepy state was not her strong suit. We couldn't get a hold of him, so at 3 a.m. she took me back to the VGH emergency room. I felt like the right side of my head was going to explode. I could feel every bone in my face and head, and then the nausea started. I threw up during the check-in process and soon found myself back in the "eye room." I pleaded with the nurses to just page the ophthalmology resident, but instead I went through a new set of ER docs who barely knew how to use the eye equipment, which didn't even work. I told them their tools weren't working and that I was in a lot of pain. They gave me an oxycodone. It did nothing, so they gave me a shot of morphine. It made me sleepy but didn't help the pain, so they gave me another shot of morphine. I fell asleep.

I was asleep for an hour or two, waking with an even more intense pain in my eye and head. Still high on morphine, I sat up to discover I was alone in the room with no call bell, but I heard my name. My friend's former girlfriend was a nurse working that night and she asked if I was okay. I said no and asked for the doctor. It turns out the eye resident had ordered an IV medication for my eye pressure, which the ER docs had been trying to get from the pharmacist for hours, but they were resistant to give it to me because it was really expensive. I was still in a lot of pain, so the ER doc gave me the eye medication and another shot of morphine. He told me it was 7:30 a.m. and the ophthalmology resident could see me down the block at the eye care center. Armed with a barf bag and in intense pain while high on morphine, my mom pushed me the two blocks to the eye center in a wheelchair.

He put some freezing drops in my eye, where he quickly poked ten times with a special pen to measure my eye pressure (I threw up twice during this stage). Normal eye pressure is around 10–15mmHg. Mine was 48mmHg. He tried to look in the eye, but it was full of blood. I couldn't see out and he couldn't see in. He said, "We are going to have to tap it." He put more freezing drops in my eye and then put a metal butterfly device into my bruised eye to hold it open. I threw up a couple more times, and then I had to rest my chin on a little ledge and stay looking down and to the left as best I could while he stuck a needle in my eye to drain some of the fluid. It was as horrible as it sounds, but it immediately eliminated the intense head pain that had been throbbing for the last twelve hours. He prescribed me an oral medication to help the pressure and sent me home for the day.

That medication became known as my zombie pills. They made me functionally useless. I spent most of the next ten days in bed, sleeping and throwing up in various levels of pain. My mother and father-in-law tried their best to get food into me, but I could only muster a few Boost vitamin drinks and a bit of yogurt, none of which I kept down. The pressure in my eye would not stabilize. I went to the eye care center every day carrying my barf bucket and ended up having my eye "tapped" with a needle seven times. I developed somewhat of a phobia of the procedure, but almost craved the relief it provided. Finally, the pressure seemed to stabilize and I started to wean off my zombie pills. The first day I went in for a check-up feeling somewhat okay, Dr. Ma tells me that the pressure is now too low, which isn't good because it can cause my retina to detach. He has me sign the paperwork for him to freeze my eye and to inject gas in attempt to raise the pressure.

This time, unfortunately, freezing didn't mean drops–it meant another needle. He froze my eye and then stuck in the needle to inject the gas. Well, I immediately returned to intense head pain and feeling nauseous. He had injected too much gas, and my pressure was back up in the 40s. *Are you kidding me?* He had to tap it again. I left feeling violated. Dr. Ma was trying his best, but my eye was not cooperating. That was a Friday. He told me to come back on Monday to follow up. I did. He was on vacation.

Enter Dr. Maberly, who was Dr. Ma's associate and, as it turns out, a high school student of my father's years earlier. I was feeling okay at this point, but I still had zero vision in my eye. It was full of blood, so I couldn't see out and he couldn't see in very well. He was concerned that my retina was detaching, but he couldn't tell for certain because he couldn't see in. He sent me for a series of eye ultrasounds over the next few days to confirm. These ultrasounds didn't hurt, but it is pretty creepy having someone move a gel-covered probe all over the surface of your eyeball. It wasn't a needle, though, so I didn't complain. After the third ultrasound on Wednesday, Dr. Maberly decided that it did look as though my retina was detaching. He pulled out the files of his patients who were scheduled for surgery the next day and had to decide which one to bump, because my eye was more urgent.

I filled out more paperwork authorizing the surgery and arrived again the next morning at VGH surgical daycare admitting. I insisted that this time they give me general anesthetic, instead of local, because the last time hurt and I was worn out from having my eye poked and prodded. I am so glad they knocked me out, because as I found out afterward, this was a "big" surgery. The resident told me in the following days that they performed nearly every possible retinal surgery on me that day. I had a vitrectomy, a scleral buckle and the insertion of another gas bubble, which meant lucky me got to lay face down for another three to five days afterward. The scleral buckle is literally a silicone band that is wrapped around the outside of my eye, which stays on forever, and it made me feel and look like I had just been punched in the face. If my eyelids were any more swollen, they would have split open.

I woke up in the recovery room to a machine beeping and a nurse encouraging me to take deeper breaths, because the oxygen saturation of my blood wasn't high enough. I was in pain and really sleepy, so it took a few hours and an oxygen mask to get me up and going. They then sent me home for my face-down sentence, part two. This one had the same result as the first one. I tolerated the position for about forty-eight hours before the pressure in my eye and face could no longer tolerate anything but laying on my side. I knew it was in the best interest of my future vision to try and stay face down, but the pain always became too much, and my mom ended up with another series of 2 a.m. phone calls to the residents.

The pressure in my eye climbed back up into the 40s, and my quality of life became inversely proportionate to that number; pain started in the 30s, nausea and intolerable pain in the 40s. My eye hurt, my head hurt more, and I was extremely nauseous. I went into the eye care center every day for the doctors to poke me in the eye and to monitor the pressure. This time, however, the docs told me that they couldn't tap it, because the relief would only last about a day—although this didn't stop them last time. The treatment of choice was to double my dosage of the zombie pills, which felt like the equivalent of giving me a frontal

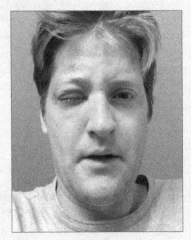

I felt about as good as I looked!

lobotomy. I slept on my mom's couch all day and stayed awake all night in pain. I discovered that if I lay on my side exactly two feet from a fan blowing on my face, it would provide mild relief, but if I got too close or stayed there too long, the bones in my face would deeply ache.

I endured the better part of a week tolerating only being horizontal, throwing up every time I rolled over. I had already missed my son's sixth birthday back in August, and now I was lining up to miss my daughter's third birthday. My wife brought the kids over to visit me on Hailey's birthday, but I could only muster sitting up for a few minutes at a time and had to rush off to throw up a few times. I didn't want them to see me like that, but I missed my family, so it was worth it.

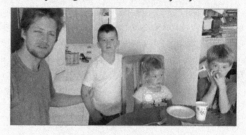

After stumbling back in to see Dr. Ma in this state, he referred me right away to a new young glaucoma doctor named Dr. Schendel. I must have looked like a homeless heroin addict when he first saw me. My hair was long, my face was gaunt with a scraggly beard and I couldn't tolerate sitting up for him to assess me. He tried his best and decided to switch my zombie pills for a different medication, instructing me to see him again in two days.

The new pills had fewer side effects, but they didn't make my eye any better. I dragged my body back to the eye care center, scaring all the old people with my barf bucket and need to lay down in the waiting room. Dr. Schendel saw me and decided we needed to do surgery that day. He worked hard to find me time in the OR and an anesthesiologist at VGH that day. In the end, he couldn't secure a time, so he admitted me through the ER so that I could get any time that came up. My mom took me to the ER on her sixty-fifth birthday, and I waited for two hours on an old dental chair, followed by three more hours on a tiny cot. Around 10:30 p.m., they brought me up to the pre-op area that I had gotten to know all too well. Again, I requested a general anesthetic, because I just needed a break from the pain.

I woke up in the recovery room, and this time I was breathing okay and I immediately felt a sense of relief. The pain in my head was gone, I wasn't nauseous, and I felt somewhat functional. The moment I had been waiting for had finally come. I was less concerned about my vision, wanting only to feel okay for the first time in a long while. I hadn't been able to keep down any food for days and hadn't drank anything the day before because I was having surgery, so I went home and enjoyed a Gatorade and a sandwich. It was amazing. Dr. Schendel had implanted an Ahmed valve on the upper-right side of my eye that has a pressure-sensitive valve inside it. If the pressure rises too high inside my eye, the valve will release fluid. It is a technology that changed my life.

I rested for one day at my mom's house before deciding it was time to move back home and be with my family. My eye and head were feeling better, but my body had an incredibly ill feeling. I had subjected it to countless amounts of Tylenol, T3s, Advil, oxycodone, morphine, zombie pills, Gravol, one local and two general anesthetics, not to mention endless vomiting. My liver, stomach and kidneys hated me, but my eye and head felt relatively better, so I was happy even though I still couldn't see very well. It was nice to be home. I read books to my kids wearing my squash goggles. I visited with my wife to try and let her know her husband was coming back. I helped walk my kids to school, which made me realize that I hadn't walked more than one hundred meters in the past two months, so three blocks felt like a marathon. I weighed myself and discovered that I had lost twenty-five pounds. I was weak, but I was home and it seemed like things were looking up.

A few days later, it was time to see Dr. Ma again. I strolled into the eye care center, and all of the staff who had so graciously helped me through the past few months individually commented on how much better I was looking. It was the first time I had shaved in a while and even remotely cared what I looked like, but it was nice to hear the positive encouragement. I felt as though I had made it through. Dr. Ma came in and looked at my eye. He said the retina and my optic nerve were looking good, but ordered a scan of the back of the eye to confirm. I don't know why, but I was actually expecting good news. As it turns out, I still had a significant hole in my macula, the center of the retina responsible for detailed vision. If this hole didn't heal, I would lose the center of my vision, and it was unlikely to heal on its own. This meant yet another surgery!

Dr. Ma kindly gave me a week to recovery from the previous three surgeries and to spend some time with my family before he went in again. That week felt like a physical vacation but a mental nightmare. I enjoyed reconnecting with my family, but I still had no functional vision for everything I had been through, and the thought of a fourth surgery was emotionally defeating. I didn't have much left in me, but it was necessary to try and save my eye. I started to feel physically better over the week, being able to eat again, which helped my confidence and mental state heading in for surgery number four. This time, he performed another vitrectomy, a membrane peel and filled my eye with a different type of gas to help me lay face down for seven days. I agreed to a local anesthetic this time and, thankfully, it didn't hurt, but it was strange listening to the doctors discuss the operation the entire time. I felt tugging, saw flashing and heard gas escaping from my eye.

The recovery from number four was a different experience than the first three. I wasn't in pain. I wasn't throwing up. It was strange for both me and my mom, who had to watch me go through it all. I moved back in with her, because I had to lay face down for an entire week, and that just doesn't work in a house with a three-, four-, and six-year-old. It was a new mental and physical challenge, but it didn't involve pain or needles in my eye, so I was up for it. I rigged a few different stations on my mom's couch and floor, and my iPhone became my entertainment center. Days were long and boring, nights were long and uncomfortable, but I did it—168 hours of looking at the floor. As soon as it was over, I moved back home and hung out with my wife and kids to try and return some normalcy to our lives.

I started enjoying life again and considered the reality of getting back to work. Three months off when you are self-employed is a very costly venture, especially when your disability insurance doesn't kick in until ninety days (I was near seventy-five). I had friends and family encouraging me to take it easy and to not rush back, but I felt up to it and wanted to get on with my life even though I still had a big gas bubble floating around in my eye. (Imagine a black marble jiggling around in the bottom of your vision as you move, and if you look down it floats up and into the center of your eye.) It was annoying and made me feel seasick as I walked, but it decreased slowly every day and finally disappeared in my third week of work. I returned to my work as a physiotherapist just under three weeks after my fourth surgery. It was a bit surreal to be back on my feet and helping other people with their pain instead of trying to deal with mine. I received amazing support from my clients, staff, and family in my return.

I am currently in week four of my return to work, and I have to say, so far so good, even though my vision is still functionally useless. I tell people that it is like looking through Tupperware: there is no acuity and plenty of double vision. The doctor says it will take about a year for the eye to heal and for my brain to more effectively use what vision I do have. In the meantime, I have four different types of medicated drops to put in my bloodshot eye throughout the day. I am not overly optimistic that full vision will return to my eye, but I have accepted that it "is what it is," and I will make the best out of it. I need to work on my depth perception, but I am comfortable driving, working and living day-to-day, so things are going to be okay. Sports have traditionally been a large part of my life, so I will have to figure out what I can and can't do, but that will happen with time. Life goes on.

**One Year Later:**
**Written August 6, 2015**

Imagine walking down the sidewalk on a nice summer day, enjoying the scenery and the sunshine all around you. Now take a visual picture of what you see and copy it. Then take that copy and paste it diagonally up and to the right and rotated slightly, so that it overlaps with half of the nice beautiful scene you are looking at. Now take that second copy and strip out all the detail and cover it with a thin layer of milky water. While you are at it, place a big smudge in the center of the picture and add distortion to anything that might be a straight line. In a sense, I now have a milky, distorted, hologram version of the world superimposed over my proper vision. And that's not even the worst part: when I walk or drive, I get the sense that the hologram world is moving at me faster than the clear, real world.

For example, every morning when I walk from my parking spot to my office, I encounter a series of tree shadows across the sidewalk and a set of two manholes. As I approach the shadows and the manholes, I see double of everything, but as I get closer and closer to the real objects, the amount of the displacement of the second blurry pictures fades to the point that they almost become one object as I pass over them. The fact that my double vision worsens the further an object is away creates the illusion that the world on the right of me is coming at me twice as fast as the world on the left, even though they are actually distorted pictures of the same thing.

My brain has tried its best to tune out the right eye, paying attention only to the left clear picture, but its capacity to do so waivers as I grow tired or move through areas where the sun is low on the horizon on my left side. Think about how difficult it can be to drive on a sunny winter morning when the sun is glaring from low in the sky. Well, I have discovered that it is quite handy to have two functional eyes in this situation instead of one, because as soon as the bright sunlight shines from the left, my brain tries to use my right eye again, until it realizes, oops, you are functionally blind in that eye! I keep both eyes open most of the time, but in situations with glaring light from the left, I am forced to shut the right and make the left endure the brightness.

When I say that I am functionally blind in my right eye, it is a difficult for most people to understand. What does that mean, exactly? It means that if I close my good eye and just look through my right one, I can see the basic layout of the room that I am in, but I can't rely on using the vision to do anything productive. I immediately feel wobbly and drunk. I cannot walk in a straight line using my right eye alone, because the damage to my macula creates an active distortion to everything that I see. I still have a hole in my macula, which has resulted in me losing the center of my vision; although I may see you standing in front of me, your face would be a brown smudge. If I wanted to see any words or letters with my right eye, I would have to hold the paper about one inch from my face and move it around to try and catch the letters with my peripheral vision.

The center of my vision is gone: the picture as a whole is now distorted and milky in nature. I have seen specialist after specialist, and one of the first things they like to do is ask me to cover my left eye and tell them what I can see on the eye chart. I have to discouragingly inform them that I can't even see the chart, and then my vision test is downgraded to "How many fingers?" at an arm's reach. It wouldn't frustrate me so much if, after every surgery, they didn't put the chart back up on the wall with the expectation that I will be able to see it, when I never have. Sad face.

People ask me why I don't wear a patch, and my answer is, "sometimes I should," and sometimes, "I do, but I have endured so much with my eye that I am not ready to give up on it yet." I close my eye when I really need to, or cover it up with my hand when the second picture is too distracting, but I believe in the neuroplasticity of the brain and the body's capacity to heal itself. I think the best chance of my eye improving is to keep using it, so I do, even though it grows tiresome every day. I wake up in the morning with a headache and go to bed every night with a different headache, but I have pushed through.

At the moment, the vision I do have in my right eye is more distracting than helpful, but I hope that over time and with one more surgery, the balance will reverse. My peripheral vision is better than my central vision, so I prefer to be aware of the objects and people to my right rather than having them disappear completely if I close my eye. Essentially, I have one-and-a-half eyes, and I hope to graduate to one-and-three-quarters, but I have no expectation of ever regaining "normal" two-eyed vision.

Thankfully, my work as a physiotherapist is accomplished more by feel than by sight. The hardest part of my day is sitting at my desk talking to clients as they tell me their story from their chair five feet away. I try my best to focus on the clear version of them on the ground as opposed to the blurry holographic version that is floating up on their left shoulder. It is tricky, and I hate it every day, but I am still holding on to hope that surgery number seven this fall may fix it. I had a fifth surgery to repair an orbital floor fracture that lifted my eyeball back up to a more normal position, but it didn't improve my vision at all; it did, however, give me six weeks of much worse headaches. The sixth surgery gave me a new lens and replaced the traumatic cataract that I developed, but so far it hasn't helped my vision, and, again, has just given me more headaches.

It is hard to not be defeated when only one of the six surgeries has yielded a positive outcome, and that wasn't even for my vision. Dr. Schendel made me a functional human being again by inserting a large tube on top of my eye to help regulate the pressure, but I have a hard time seeing a silver lining in any of the other five so far. I am placing a lot of hope in my last surgery and genuinely cannot wait to be done with interventions so that I can move past hope and actually mourn the loss that I have suffered.

Last October, after my fourth surgery in two months, the best I could get out of Dr. Ma was, "What you need is about a year. Your eye will heal and your brain will figure out how to better use what it's got." Well, it has been about a year and I apparently needed more than just time, because I've had two more surgeries and am on the wait list for another that should round things out at an uneven seven surgeries and a countless number of "procedures."

As I approach the one-year anniversary of my eye injury, I am finding myself spending more and more time reflecting on the impact it has had on my life and that of my family. I have tried my best to move forward, but almost a year later I find the whole incident still playing a central role in my day-to-day life. I have returned to full-time work as a physiotherapist, business owner, father of three young children, husband, and semi-professional visitor of eye doctors. Our life didn't have room for this to happen, but it did and we have had to figure out how to make it work.

After returning to work, I discovered the unique challenge of working as a physiotherapist trying to help people in pain when, all along, they know what I have recently been through. After twelve years as a physiotherapist, I have an incredibly sympathetic and caring clientele that is concerned about my well-being. I am grateful for this, but recapping my story and current status with a new person every thirty minutes all day has been one of my greatest mental challenges. I am not used to being the focus of so many people's sympathy, and it is extremely hard to remain positive when you have to tell a depressing story fourteen times a day. Most people ask about my prognosis with the expectation that my sight will return. I have to be the one to say, "Well, it's not looking like it, but I still have a few more surgeries to go." Leading up to each surgery, we get to talk about the prospects of its success, but afterward I get to share my disappointment that it didn't really help and receive more pity and sympathy. The physical battle has been tough, but the mental challenge has been a more complex beast to handle.

I know I have a loss to mourn, but the way this injury has panned out, almost a year later I still don't know what exactly I have lost because I am on the wait list for surgery number seven. I am still in it. It is an acute phase that just won't end, because there is always another surgery. After my recent cataract surgery failed to restore any acuity of vision, I have started coming to terms with the loss of the functional vision in my right eye. That said, I am still holding on to hope that my distracting and fatiguing double vision can be improved.

Everything is harder now. I can still do most things, but most of them are more difficult than they once were. The first question most people ask me is, "Can you still drive?" The answer is, "Yes, I can still drive, but parking is a challenge." My depth perception for cars behind me when I'm parallel parking is compromised, but I am learning to adapt. The world on the right of me coming at me at double speed is distracting, but I am learning to adapt. Coaching my five-year-old's baseball team was hard, but I'm getting better at catching balls. Pouring juice into a glass and inserting a key into a keyhole continue to challenge, but I'm figuring them out. One day I hope to settle into my new normal, but for now I try my best to endure the exhausting process of figuring out a new strategy for the little things in life.

I wake up every morning with a mild headache and a dry, irritated, goopy cornea. I spend the first five minutes tending to my eye at the bathroom sink. It doesn't feel somewhat comfortable until I have had a shower, and even then it still feels as though I have something in my eye. Over the past year, I have gone through periods of time where I was on up to four different medicated drops that needed to be put in one to four times a day each; thankfully, I am now down to one glaucoma drop at bedtime, but I am still required to use a thick tear gel five to six times a day to keep my dry eye somewhat comfortable. I get occasional short but strong pains in my eye throughout the day and typically develop a gripping headache up the right side of my head by the end of a workday. Thankfully, the more time since my most recent surgery, the less painful and frequent my headaches become. I make the best of every day, because I enjoy my job, I love my family and I believe that life holds too much fun to be ruined by pain.

If you need any more incentive to wear eye protection while playing sports, consider my list of injuries from one backhand shot in a pick-up ball hockey game:

- Detached retina (two surgeries)

- Macular hole (two surgeries)

- Orbital floor fracture (one surgery)

- My iris is stuck in a dilated position (forced to live with it!)

- Inability to regulate the pressure in my eye without my new valve (one surgery + seven needles in my eye)

- My two eyes don't point in the same direction anymore = double vision (surgery upcoming)

- Traumatic cataract (one surgery)

This experience has helped me develop wisdom, courage, empathy and perseverance. It has replaced some of my confidence with vulnerability and given me more compassion for people who face real challenges in their lives. I have been knocked down a peg by this ordeal, but I plan on coming out the other side with a new perspective on the world and with my head held high.

One more to go!

**My Final Surgery:**
**Written March 2016**

So, is this what my vision is going to be like for the rest of my life? On the other side of seven surgeries, I now have to live with the product of six surgeons' expertise and my brain's ability to adapt. My eyeball is permanently wrapped in a band of silicone, supported by a piece of mesh, pressure regulated by a large tube, "focuses" with an artificial lens and is held in alignment by newly attached muscles. So far, my retina has stayed in place, and my cornea continues to be irritated about the entire experience. I have literally seen every sub-specialty of ophthalmology and am not sure that I am further ahead than if I had permanently lost the vision in my right eye a year and a half ago.

I find myself entering the new mental challenge of trying to be happy about the moderate success of my last surgery and the fact that I am "done," while at the same time coming to the realization that I must go through the rest of my life with significantly compromised vision. Esthetically, my last surgery made me look normal again, which is significant. My right eye had been pulled in and down toward my nose, but thanks to Dr. Lyons my two eyes now largely point in the same direction. Under general anesthetic, he released the muscle attachments on either side of my eye, repositioned it based on their measurements and then reattached them in a new position. I woke up in the recovery room with a giant letter "E" on a post at the foot of my bed and the doctor asking me, "So, how is it now?" If I didn't say "good," they were going to knock me out again and readjust the eye.

I didn't say "good"; instead, I said in a groggy voice, "Now the second 'E' is over there," pointing to my left. My double vision had been separated diagonally up and right, whereas now it seemed less up, but definitely to the left. He overshot it the other way. He asked for my feedback, but decided that he had done the best he could and said that the tube prevented him from adjusting it any further. So now it is what it is until either technology makes me a cyborg or stem cell treatment for the eyes becomes a reality. For now, I am just happy to have doctors no longer poking away in there, and I am looking forward to the time when people's first question for me is something other than "How's your eye?"

I discovered a few months before my last surgery, after enduring double vision for over a year in attempt to let my brain try to adapt, that putting Scotch tape on a pair of glasses to make the right lens opaque made my vision much more comfortable. It allowed me to keep the eye open and allow light in, but it took the second "picture" away and made for a much more relaxing visual experience. It was more comfortable, but as with everything I changed, it gave me more headaches for a while.

After my last surgery, I found that I had more tolerance for my new form of double vision than my old form, but I still found myself putting my ghetto glasses back on by lunchtime and to work on the computer. I'm not a very self-conscious person, but wearing a visual reminder of my injury on my face is a frustrating dilemma. My eye now looks largely normal, but my vision is still one notch below useful, so wearing my taped-up glasses helps my vision, but also triggers everyone else to comment or ask about my eye, making it more difficult to move on. Time will help the mental aspect of it, but the knowledge that nothing can help my actual vision is something that I am still getting used to.

# Why Heads Hurt

After reading the previous section, you may have a better understanding about where my headaches come from, but it did not likely shed much light on your experiences. Headaches have many sources and attack in a number of forms: migraines, neck tension, behind your eyes, in your temples, and so on. Your head has the capacity to mildly and chronically hurt for years and even lay you out in a dark room for two-day stints of torture.

Most people's first response to a headache is to swallow a magic pill that takes the edge off by generally treating their symptom with a medicinal bomb to their physiology. Headaches are a significant industry for the pharmaceutical companies, because they can usually offer some quick relief and allow a person to be functional at little cost or effort. The trouble with effectively treating the symptom and ignoring the cause is that the side effects of the drugs start to become just as bad as the headache and can compound the original problem. I have had some form of headache or another every day since I injured my eye, so believe me when I say that I understand that Advil can be a necessary evil. If you really want to stop or lessen your pattern of pill consumption, though, start looking into other options that address your body as a whole.

The root cause of a headache is not normally in the head itself but a combination of factors including stress, posture, alignment, mechanical tension, and organ mobility. Our emotional state and our organs are intimately connected with each other, which can be reflected in both our posture and our alignment. When you feel sad, you may literally feel a heaviness in your heart. When you are nervous, you may feel "butterflies" in your stomach. When you are angry, you might feel a strong visceral reaction, likely around your liver. If you are anxious, your G.I. tract may act up. All of these emotional reactions can and do create mechanical tension in your body and have the capacity to affect your head.

Organs need to be able to move around to properly do their job, allowing you to be healthy and mobile. Your body will do a great job to accommodate and protect their function by tensing up certain muscles in response to fascial strains on the organs, which can result in persistent alignment problems. If a therapist only treats the muscular and bony outer shell of a person to get them back in alignment, the results may be short-lived if an organ-emotion is the underlying driver of the problem. Understanding your own mind-body connection is an important part of controlling and minimizing your recurrent headaches, as is finding a therapist with the capacity to consider the role of your container and its contents in treating your headache.

Headaches are not purely an emotional problem. Mechanical tension on your head and body can arise from ergonomic issues, jarring injuries, and invasive surgeries that create strain on your muscles, nerves, blood vessels, organs and the web of connective tissue that holds it all together. Tension can come from almost anywhere in your body and still affect your head. Imagine if I had you wear a full spandex suit and then grabbed a handful of the material near the front of your right hip and pulled down; you would feel it tugging on your upper body and head. This concept happens throughout your body in three-dimensional planes as you move around, and it can be a negative consequence of how connected everything is. The surgery on your bladder may have created a downward tug. Your body may still be bracing your side after your kidney infection. Everything you have experienced in the past plays a role in how you feel now, so be open to considering your past medical history even if you don't think it is relevant to your current issue.

Your neck, spine, and brain are particularly vulnerable to whiplash forces from behind and jarring forces like falling on your tailbone or hip. These types of trauma have the capacity to deeply irritate your nervous system and, as a result, create a great deal of compressive tension in your muscular system. It is like having too many amps running through your circuits until somebody helps your body figure out how to calm itself. Your overly-excited nervous system can create bands of tension in large areas of muscle and irritability in your organs. Tension in your muscles, nerves, and organs will commonly find its way into giving you a headache.

Your brain is wrapped in a protective lining called the dura. It extends down your brain stem, around your spinal cord, and anchors in the middle of your sacrum just above your tailbone. In order for you to bend forward in your neck and upper back, your dura needs to be able to slide and stretch upward in the spinal column. Conversely, in order for you to flex forward through your hips and lower back, your dura needs to be able to slide and stretch downward. You can end up with a tug-of-war happening between the base of your skull and your tailbone through your dura. It is closely connected to your eyes and is affected by the attachments of your organs to the back wall of your abdominal and thoracic cavities. Dural tension is a common culprit involved in chronic headaches, and because the dura is intimately connected to your nervous system—the connector of everything—tension in one area can get transmitted to your head through the dura.

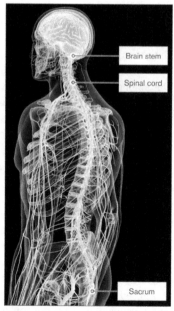

Brain stem

Spinal cord

Sacrum

Dura is the protective lining around your brain and extends down your brain stem, around your spinal cord, to the middle of your sacrum.

Through the process of learning the manual skill of what osteopath Jean-Pierre Barral calls neuromeningeal manipulation (NM, a technique comparable to cranio-sacral therapy), I have come to appreciate the importance of the mobility of the bones and membranes in the skull and face. You can develop torsions and tension patterns in your head in the same way you can in your pelvis, and often the two are related. Your temporal bones right behind your ears can torsion similar to your pelvis, and tend to be a reflection of tension in a membrane that supports your brain called the tentorium. The tentorium is commonly strained in whiplash and jarring accidents and can be the driving force behind problems down one side of the body. Another important area is the junction of where the bones of your face meet the bones of your skull. People will commonly experience torsions in this joint after blows to the face, dental procedures, or grinding their teeth, and it can be reflected in the palate of the mouth. Cranial torsions can directly cause headaches and jaw problems and indirectly create problems elsewhere in the body through the strong connection of the dura.

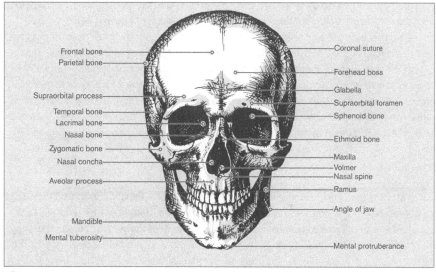

Diagram of the cranial bones and skull.

I have found that the best way to clinically treat headaches is to begin with a thorough assessment of a person's posture and alignment, followed by listening to where the strongest pull in the body is coming from; sometimes it is the head, sometimes it's not. If it is the head, I will start with manually trying to ease any tension using NM, and then try to further calm the nervous system and muscular tension in the body with intramuscular stimulation on the neck, spine and hips. I've experienced success in combining these two treatment modalities, but I often had to incorporate visceral manipulation, postural retraining, and cognitive awareness into the mix to properly get the headaches under control. Everyone's body has its own story, and the more options your therapist has to solve your three-dimensional moving puzzle, the more likely you will find a positive outcome.

# The Cumulative Effect: You are the Product of Everything You Have Done, Seen, and Experienced up to This Moment

When pain seemingly comes out of nowhere or appears disproportionate to the activity that brought it on, people always want to know what it was they did wrong to end up in pain. If they could go back in time and change that one movement, their pain would be erased forever. Pain can make you very short-sighted if you have a need to place blame on one event to justify what is happening. I try to open people's eyes to the idea that just because their body didn't hurt last week like it does now, doesn't mean that everything was working perfectly. There is a lot going on in the body every second of every day of which we are not aware, but pain and injuries have a way of drawing attention to the areas that need a tune-up. Some people are more body aware than others and can sense when something isn't feeling right and proactively have it looked at before it becomes a bigger problem. Most people, however, ignore the warning signs and wait until the engine light comes on and smoke billows out of the hood before they seek out help.

The history of pain and dysfunction in any person's body is usually a long and entangled story, of which the person is only partly aware. People will focus on the car accidents, sports injuries, or surgeries, but they gloss over the problem areas that they can't blame on someone else, like how they stand, sit, walk, and breathe all day, or the amount of stress in their lives. The body has an incredible capacity to heal from acute injuries, but it has a more trying time dealing with the day-in, day-out micro-traumas we put our bodies through by moving poorly, sitting for hours at a time, eating junk food and living stressful lives. Your body does have a breaking point, and typically when pain starts insidiously, whatever you did just before it started was likely just the "straw that broke the camel's back" and not the activity that deserves all the blame. Pain can result from your bad habits catching up to you, and it offers a time for self-reflection.

Although our bodies do heal, our tissues and our brains have a memory for the traumas that they have been through and can subconsciously affect how you move and feel. Our bodies will often compensate for one restricted area by moving in another to alleviate the pain, but that only works until the compensation starts causing something else to start hurting. The role of physiotherapy is not to only to relieve the pain, but help your body to make sense of the traumas it has sustained, both mentally and

physically to minimize the chain of events that can occur. In many cases, /
into physiotherapy already deep into a chain of events that may have be
years earlier when they sprained their ankle or got rear-ended. The acute pu.
with time, but the dysfunction continued and fell below their radar long enough to
create problems elsewhere in their body. Old ankle sprains are the root cause of many
back and pelvis problems, as are old, mild whiplash injuries responsible for persistent
hip problems. The interconnection of all the systems in your body helps to create
redundancies and back-up strategies to keep you mobile, but it can also create a
complex web to untangle for some people in getting out of pain.

The more I improve at neural manipulation, the more I realize that persistent foot and
ankle problems tend to be rooted in torsions in the upper back and base of the skull.
Twisting tension patterns from old whiplash injuries, blows to the head, and even a
good deal of dental work commonly irritate the dura, the protective lining of the brain
and spinal cord, and can refer tension almost anywhere in the body; quite often this is
the cause of shin and heel pain. When the ankle becomes locked up from dural tension,
it doesn't allow a person to squat well, and activities like running will result in a jammed
ankle, creating a torsion in the pelvis as a compensation. In short, you can seemingly
do everything right, but your past may come back to haunt you in unexpected ways. It
takes some explaining by me—and trust by my clients—when they come in with a sore
ankle and I start fiddling with their mouth and neck, but the tensions in the body tell a
story of your past that you don't always remember. A good manual therapist can likely
feel what you can't see.

Different events in your life will trigger a variety of emotions based on your past
experiences. Many people who were in bad car accidents have stress related to driving,
and the simple act of getting into the car can trigger recurrent pains. Different emotions
are often held as tension in different organs and can manifest as pain after triggering
events. I have witnessed plenty of truth to what osteopath Jean-Pierre Barral discussed
in his book Understanding the Messages of Your Body. I've started to see and feel that
common areas of restriction in people's bodies often correlate to certain personality
traits. The lens through which you see the world affects the physical characteristics of
your body and your pain. "Type A" people may wonder why they can have much more
difficulty with a yoga pose than the person beside them, even though they are trying
hard; contrary to their lens, success isn't always about the quantity of effort.

I find perspective to be a funny thing as it relates to pain, because some people have
none. It is foreign to me that a person can get all the way into their mid-forties without
truly hurting themselves, but those people are out there and you'd think it was the end
of the world when they come in with a sore back. After three days of pain, they often
have this sense of panic that they will remain this way forever, or think that they are
going to need surgery. Sometimes a lack of experience with your body can make one
minor injury have as negative of an effect as having experienced several minor injuries.
Hurting yourself helps you build a relationship with your body to help you understand

what is and isn't normal, and it teaches you not to panic, because time often fixes minor problems.

I speak from experience when I talk about the cumulative effect, having witnessed and lived it both professionally and personally. I have treated four generations of the same family in my office and have seen the nature-versus-nature phenomenon in the individuals' body types, personalities, and history of injuries over a ninety-year age span. I have also learned a lot about myself and my body by treating both of my parents, my wife, and my three children. All of my family's behavior as it relates to pain and injury is affected by my being a physiotherapist with a long history of injuries. My ability to endure the relentless medical procedures, surgeries, and doctor appointments related to my eye injury was profoundly affected by my familiarity with doctors and hospitals, but I can imagine the experience could have created a post-traumatic stress disorder in someone less comfortable with the medical system.

If you feel stuck in a maze when dealing with your persistent pain problem, consider your past physical, emotional, and social experiences as contributing factors, and be open to dealing with more than just your immediate pain.

> *"What you are is what you have been. What you'll be is what you do now."*
> *–Buddha*

# Diane Lee's Story: Mom, Physiotherapist, Woman

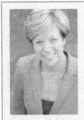

Diane Lee graciously agreed to tell her story for the purpose of this book. The following article offers words of wisdom from a world-class physiotherapist, who happened to develop a resistant pain problem in her area of specialty, and the journey it took her down. Enter Diane . . .

www.DianeLee.ca

As a patient, what gets done to you depends on what story you tell and who you tell it to. As a physiotherapist, what you do depends on what patients tell you and how you interpret their stories. As a mom and a woman, you suck it up and "soldier on." I am all those "people" and here is my story.

I am a 61-year-old mother of two and a physiotherapist. In 2012, I took a teacher training course in Anusara yoga, and during this course I came to realize that my left hip was somewhat stiffer than my right, but didn't think much about it; after all, I was in my late '50s and it didn't hurt, it was just stiff.

In 2014, I fainted at 40,000 feet in the air (in an airplane) and landed on my left side. I hurt my collar bone and shoulder, and over time with the right physiotherapy it has healed quite nicely. Four months after this fall, though, I started to wake in the night with a deep ache, sometimes in the left buttock, sometimes in my left groin, sometimes in my left inner thigh. On occasion, the muscles on the inside of my thigh would cramp or spasm and seriously make me jump out of bed. The pain and cramps would cease within seconds of sitting up, but, of course, you can't sleep all night sitting up!

Over the next six months I wasn't able to sleep more than three hours without getting up, and, of course, once you wake up in the middle of the night you go to the bathroom—why not, you're awake. What I began to realize over time was that voiding (peeing) would also relieve my hip pain. Now that was strange to me. At this time, I didn't have any pain during the day and my ability to do yoga, train, walk, etc., wasn't being impacted; I was just becoming sleep deprived.

In 2015, one year after the fall in the airplane, the ache began to present when I was vertical, during the day. People started to ask me, "Why are you limping?" It had all started so gradually that I didn't notice I was. Over time I lost a lot of hip extension and internal rotation, two movements you need in order to walk well. My yoga practice made the night pain worse, and I had stopped all training in the gym. I was starting to notice increasing difficulty breathing when I spoke for long periods of time. I talk a lot for my job and this was an increasing problem.

I began conservative treatment. I had it all: physiotherapy, massage, chiropractic, and visceral treatment from some of the world's best clinicians, because I know a lot of them. I even had internal pelvic-floor work done, thinking that the nerves to my hip must be a problem on the inside since nothing on the outside was working. When one of the nerves to my hip (obturator nerve) was touched, it totally reproduced my hip pain and flared all of my pain for days. Clearly the obturator nerve was a pain generator, but what was causing the irritation of the nerve? I kept looking for someone to "release the internal vector that was pulling on the nerve." While everything helped temporarily, nothing helped for long and eventually nothing helped at all.

By November 2015, I could only walk one block without developing a significant limp, I couldn't sleep without being somewhat propped up with my hip flexed, and breathing was a real struggle. And still, voiding at night gave some relief. Why was I hurting? A friend and colleague who chairs a World Congress on pelvic pain was visiting from Europe, and when we were walking on Crescent Beach one afternoon, he said "Lee, why are you limping?" I told him a brief version of my hip story–not the entire story–and related it all to the fall on the airplane a year and a half prior. He said, "You have to push back, this is your nervous system, your brain is creating the pain, push back or you will be a cripple!" This is the latest evidence from the neuroscience in chronic pain. "There is nothing wrong in the tissue; your brain is in a state of threat and makes you think you are damaging yourself by moving, but you really aren't." So, I pushed back and tried to do exercises in order to increase my hip mobility every morning. It made the pain during the day and night worse.

I became the patient on a mission to find out "what's wrong with me?" and "why am I hurting?" I was confident that this wasn't in my brain. Finally, at the end of November 2015, I brought out my own ultrasound imaging machine that I use as a physiotherapist to train core strategies for the abdominal wall and pelvic floor, and saw something on my uterus that I had forgotten about.

Twelve years ago I started on a bio-identical hormone replacement program for menopause, which includes bio-identical estrogen supplements. I love my estrogen. Uterine fibroids love estrogen too, and usually after menopause they shrink, but in my case, because I continued to feed it estrogen, they grew. In fact, one had grown a lot. It had first been discovered when I had a pelvic ultrasound at age fifty-three (just for prevention purposes before starting a hormone program), but it was small and not creating any problems (or so I thought), so I left it alone. And in the twelve years since then, it kept growing and growing, enlarging the back wall on the right side of my uterus.

In early December 2015, I paid privately to have a total-body MRI to get a clear image of the fibroid and more information about my lower back and left hip. The hip pain story I was telling everyone could be due to degeneration of my lower back, osteoarthritis of my left hip, or maybe—just maybe (but it's not usual I was told)—from the fibroid pulling on the internal fascia and irritating the left obturator nerve (my hypothesis). The MRI showed all three problems: severe degeneration at L2-3 (where the obturator nerve comes from) with a disc protrusion compressing the nerve roots, mild to moderate osteoarthritis of my left hip, and a big fibroid pushing my sacrum backward.

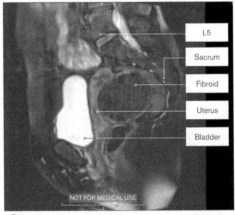

MRI of the pelvic area showing uterine fibroid.

When you pay privately for an MRI, you are given thirty minutes with the radiologist who reviews the findings with you: fabulous idea. I told him I was a physiotherapist and may have some different questions than usual and thanked him for being patient with my questions as I tried to understand my hip pain better. As he scanned down my whole-body MRI, he stopped in my lower back and showed me some damage at L2-3 and said, "Here is your problem. You should have a microdiscectomy here." I explained, "I was a competitive gymnast when I was young and experienced lots of compression loading in my spine. 20% of so-called positive findings on MRI are inaccurate, or false, for explaining current pain conditions. I'm wondering why peeing in the middle of the night is what gives me pain relief if this disc is the problem." He replied, "What? I've never heard of that. No, that wouldn't be from your disc, but I have more!" If I didn't tell him about the peeing part of my story and left it as hip pain during the night, I might have ended up with unnecessary surgery on my back. The "more" was the huge fibroid on the back of my uterus and arthritis in my left hip. I noticed on the MRI that the angle of my sacrum was very horizontal, and that was consistent with how my standing posture had changed over the last year and a half. I could not stand without sticking my butt out backward and increasing the curve in my lower back.

I had seen enough from this MRI to be convinced that the arthritis in my hip was being caused by over-activation of the hip muscles supplied by this irritated nerve that caused excessive compression of my hip into the socket. These muscles externally rotate and flex the hip, thus my limitation of hip extension (leg going behind you), internal rotation, and limp. I was beginning to understand "why I was hurting."

If I lifted what I thought was my uterus/fibroid in my low pelvis, my hip motion would improve and immediately worsen when I let it go. OK, now we're onto something! But what to do? What were my options? I consulted more doctors, and here is what I was told, as I told a slightly different story to each of them:

1. Uterine fibroids.:These are more often a problem to women in their thirties who still want to have children. They can cause excessive bleeding, and this is usually the main symptom. I had no uterine bleeding. In this group, a medication is given to inhibit estrogen, which results in shrinkage of the fibroid. This wouldn't work for me, because I wanted to stay on my estrogen (for healthy brain aging). To go off the estrogen and wait months for the fibroid to shrink may mean a happy hip but also for sure an unhappy, foggy, forgetful brain. Furthermore, if I started the estrogen again, the fibroid would merely grow back after a period of time and I would be back to square one—maybe. This clearly wasn't a great option.

2. Uterine artery embolization: In this procedure, they essentially cut off the blood flow to the fibroid (and in my case, the uterus) to "kill it." It was described to me like having a "heart attack in your pelvis." You would be hospitalized for three to five days of agony, and then your uterus/fibroid would be dead and maybe it would shrink 20%. Really? If the mass was the problem (the fibroid wasn't bleeding), how would this help reduce the nerve tension and the consequences it was causing to my hip? No thanks.

3. Hysterectomy (taking out the mass): There are a few ways to remove a uterus and many consequences when this is not done right. I know because, as a physiotherapist, I treat women with post-hysterectomy complications. This seemed to be the best option if I could convince the right surgeon about how I wanted this done.

I am very fortunate to work with two open, curious, and intelligent OB-GYNs who both saw me, at my request, for advice. Neither thought my situation was "usual," and one offered me the "ten-minute vaginal hysterectomy" which I rejected. I had developed a postpartum rectocele many years ago which I managed well conservatively. What is a rectocele? It is a weakening of the posterior part of the vagina that then allows the rectum to bulge into it. There is no tear—just stretching—but it makes having a bowel movement difficult at times. The idea of pulling anything out my vagina didn't make sense to me. The second surgeon had a better idea. He had a colleague OB-GYN who was recently trained in "minimally invasive laparoscopic" hysterectomies. He suggested inviting her to do the uterine/fibroid removal while he repaired the rectocele. I met her, liked her a lot, and decided to go with it. Both had never heard of fibroids causing limited range of motion of the hip and night pain, but when I showed them how my standing posture and hip mobility changed when I lifted my uterus/fibroid, they were convinced.

Surgery was booked for one month later—I got lucky in our Canadian medical system to have this done so quickly. Immediately after surgery, while in the recovery room, I could feel that the internal vector that for years had been pulling on my hip was gone. My left leg lay in full extension with ease. I couldn't completely rotate it internally, but I had known during pre-op that there would likely be some physiotherapy necessary post-op in order to get back to full function.

And that's where I'm at now. Post-op recovery, twenty-two days. Guidelines: no lifting anything heavier than ten pounds for four weeks. I have not had any surgical pain in my abdominal wall, nor my pelvis area since one week after the surgery. It would be very tempting to ignore the surgeon's directions of no lifting more than ten pounds IF I didn't have the ability to use ultrasound imaging to witness my healing. I have no pain—I repeat, no pain—but I can see on the ultrasound that the fascia they cut through to gain access to my uterus/fibroid is not healed. It would be easy to get back into some "gentle yoga," but that would strain the fascia. You can't do much without your abdominal wall contracting. Imagine a cut on your knuckle. Every time you bend it too much, it cracks open and healing has to start all over again. If I load my trunk too much (lift the dogs, vacuum, push heavy doors, etc.), I have to use my abdominal muscles as well as my pelvic floor. If I exceed the healing limit, things just may come undone or start to hurt. 30% of laparoscopic surgeries have some degree of hernia post-op. Pain is a representation of threat at this stage of healing. As long as I don't threaten my tissue, it will continue to heal.

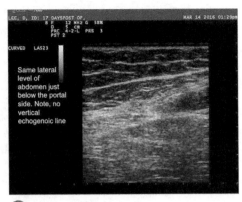

⬆ Normal abdominal muscles.

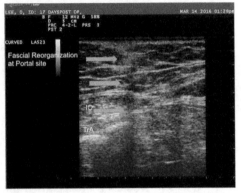

⬆ One of the 'portals' where they cut through my abdomen; this shows the fascial reorganization.

As my husband said when I was getting antsy and had not assessed myself yet with the ultrasound, "You have the rest of your life to get going, now is the time to rest."

My message: tell your whole story, every bit of it. You have no idea how connected everything is, so don't leave out something you think may not matter. Take control of your own therapy and medical investigations, and get as much knowledge as you can. It is empowering, and trust that the answer lies in your story. I'm very happy that I can explain "why I hurt" and that I am on the path to not hurting, and leading an active life once again.

# Take Aways and Resources

## Take Aways

→ Health professionals who step into another person's journey need to appreciate that everybody approaches the world through their own lens, and has their own relationship with pain.

→ Pain is a product of integrated systems and should be treated that way.

→ IMS (intramuscular stimulation) is an extremely powerful and important tool that can be used to calm down the nervous system and treat chronic pain.

→ Restrictions in the mobility of your organs can be the root cause of your alignment and pain problems.

→ Mental awareness of your body and mind is an essential life skill to develop.

→ You are a product of everything you have done, seen, and experienced up to this moment.

→ Wear eye protection when playing sports!

## Websites

✚ BarralInstitute.com: Osteopath Jean-Pierre Barral's curriculum of visceral and neural manipulation courses.

✚ DianeLee.ca: Physiotherapist and co-creator of the Integrated Systems Model.

✚ iSTOP.org: Physician Dr. Chan Gunn, creator of intramuscular stimulation (IMS).

✚ DrDanSiegel.com: Psychiatrist and author of Mindsight.

✚ WhyThingsHurt.com: Resources that integrate the knowledge of the above three.

# Fitness, Exercise, and Sports

## Myths to Dispel:

- You are stiff because you didn't stretch enough

- Strengthening exercises are always helpful

- More exercise is always better than less

# How Sports Affect Your Body Throughout Life

*"We are what we repeatedly do. Excellence, then, is not an act, but a habit."*
*—Aristotle*

For many of us, sports become a part of who we are, both mentally and physically. For children, sports are a means of socializing, but they also play a prominent role in the development of movement. For adults, sports become a means of fitness, stress relief, competition and, commonly, injury. No matter where you find yourself on the spectrum of young to old, or novice to professional, sports have likely impacted your body in some way. Appreciating how, and to what extent, may help you address chronic problems, prevent future ones, and will likely maximize your performance.

Each sport comes with its own particular set of movement patterns required of its athletes. Dancers have chest up, shoulders down, butt clenched, and toes out drilled into them. Tennis players and golfers spend hours twisting one way and not the other. Bikers ride hundreds of miles with their bodies tucked into a tight aerodynamic position with their head poking up, and runners get used to going straight forward all the time. How much these movement experiences will affect you depend on what stage of your life you do them in, how much you do them, and whether you play a variety of other sports or have committed to the performance of just one.

Early movement experiences mold a child's posture and coordination for later in life, which is why I encourage physical play with my kids. Activities like chase, wrestling, rolling, jumping, throwing, and catching help kids build an awareness of how to use their bodies. They get some bumps and bruises along the way, but it helps them learn that pain is temporary and that their bodies are amazing at healing themselves if they give them a chance. As a physiotherapist, I can quickly tell the difference between adults who have a physical, athletic history, and ones who have led a fairly sedentary lifestyle, both in their body awareness and their outlook on their current pain or dysfunction. Past athletes tend to have a more optimistic and in-control attitude about their rehabilitation, because they have fostered relationships with their bodies due to past experience. Conversely, adults who haven't competed in sports in their youth tend to be much less assertive in their healing and much more dependent on health professionals, because they are less in tune with their bodies.

Although athletes are more in tune with their bodies, they tend to develop posturally with strong imbalances based on their sport of choice. Dancers and figure skaters get swaybacks and bad hips. Tennis players, golfers, and volleyball players get left-right asymmetries. They all experience the world through the body and lens of the athlete they are, but, unfortunately, only the rare few turn their sport into their career, and what might help them in sport might hinder them in life. When you tune your body so finely to do one activity, it can make other tasks—like work—more difficult and even painful. Loosey-goosey dancers have a hard time staying posturally still at desk jobs. Asymmetrical golfers can experience trouble when bending and lifting, because their backs can be vulnerable. It can go both ways: pain and performance issues in sport can be rooted in ergonomic, postural issues at work, and chronic tension and pain at work can be a result of the strong muscle imbalances developed in sport. We are what we repeatedly do.

People who have devoted a lot of their time to elite, sport-specific training are a fun group to treat, because they can appreciate the nuances of how small corrections to their body position can significantly improve their performance; it isn't a huge mental leap for them to understand that subtle changes in their posture and movement might relieve their pain. That being said, they can have further trouble changing their movement patterns, because they excel at moving the way they do, and it can be harder to learn something new when it doesn't fit into the mold they have created with their training. People who develop their bodies into finely-tuned instruments for one activity become vulnerable to injury when you ask them to try something else, which is why cross-training can be very important for some athletes.

I broadly categorize people into three groups: elite athletes (past and present), multi-sport/ "jack-of-all-trades" athletes, and non-athletes. The elite group is the most fun to work with, the multi-sport group is the easiest, and the non-athletes are the most challenging but also the most rewarding. Elite athletes tend to be fast learners and are keen to push themselves, but have to work through their imbalances. Jack-of-all-trades athletes are body aware and have less bias, but they may have a history of more injuries due to increased exposure to a variety of strenuous activities. Finally, non-athletes tend to be what I call "motor morons," where simple movement exercises can baffle them, because they have never considered how to move before; their bodies are simply vehicles with which to move their heads around.

Everyone starts out as a small child just trying to move and is gradually filtered into one of my three broad groups over time; which group an individual ends up in will likely determine how sports will affect their body as an aging adult. I like to call it the "Goldilocks Phenomenon," in regards to the amount of sport and exercise that is appropriate for a person while they are aging. Everyone has a personal level of how much exercise is too much, too little, or "just right," but the conscious mind's "just right" is not always the same as the physical body's. I need to motivate some people to do more, some I have to convince to do less, and some just need reassurance that they are in the "just right" part of their curve.

Aging athletes commonly require guidance on balancing activity and recovery time in any given week. Their brain may want to play tennis four days a week, but their body maxes out at three, and anything beyond that creates pain and injuries. I encourage older clients to find what author Tim Ferriss calls their "minimal effective dose" of exercise and sports; what is the least they can do in a week that will provide the most benefits, both physically and mentally? Older people also tend to be creatures of habit and hold the same exercise regimes for years or even decades, so I like to introduce variety and create awareness of the idea that their body doesn't stay the same year to year, so neither should their level of exercise.

Many non-athletes tend to take up exercising later in life when they feel the need to lose weight or "get in shape." The two most common choices seem to be running and weight lifting, because the barrier to entry for the activity is quite low. The aspect that most adults in this group fail to recognize is that these activities require skilled movement to perform correctly and to not cause injury. Any able-bodied person can run, but to do it regularly and for long distances requires skill to not hurt themselves. The same is true for weight lifting: pushing, pulling, and heavy lifting will likely make you stronger, but it requires skill to do it regularly without hurting yourself. The non-athletes tend to jump into new activities by focusing on the new activity itself rather than learning how to do it properly. I ask my clients to start with very basic movement exercises and have them earn the right to progress further. A non-athlete may take six months to progress to where their more body-aware counterpart could advance in two weeks. If they take the time to learn how their body moves doing small exercises, their fitness won't plateau or fall off a cliff due to injury.

In an ideal world, children would start developing body awareness through a variety of fun sports and games from the ages of three to eighteen years old, but, unfortunately, physical education has taken the back burner to academics in most school systems, and kids are left to figure out their bodies by themselves. I believe a system that could teach the fundamentals of athleticism to young children would be hugely beneficial to our society, because the only way to create a truly preventative healthcare system is to educate the people on how to use their bodies from a young age. Physical movement creates an appreciation of body awareness in people, as well as a sense of what is normal or abnormal in their bodies. People who are in tune with their "normal" selves take care of their bodies, and know when to reach out for help. People who don't create a physical relationship with their body from a young age tend to be more unhealthy and create strain on our healthcare system later in life.

Sports should be viewed as more than just play, but also as an opportunity to learn and be healthy, at any age. People need to appreciate where they are on the growth and development curve to realize just how much their sport of choice may be affecting them. School kids are growing and developing while they are playing the most sports, so, like it or not, their teenage years may define some of their physical future. Adults over the age of thirty begin their march toward stenosis and need to appreciate that, despite their best efforts, their body is slowly degenerating and requires a bit more maintenance to keep going than it once did.

My advice:

1. Play with your kids from a young age.

2. Expose your kids to many different sports instead of trying to build a professional athlete at a young age.

3. Acknowledge your diminishing invincibility while heading into your thirties and adjust your lifestyle.

4. Stay active every day, but appreciate the value of rest days; find your minimal effective dose.

5. Think of your aging body as an aging car: you can still push it to its limits, as long as you have learned to drive it well and put in the time and effort to maintain it.

# Pole Dancers, MMA Fighters, and Cirque Performers: Balancing Pain and Elite Performance

My favorite part of being a physiotherapist is the glimpses I am given into other people's worlds, especially the worlds of athletes. I have always been a jack-of-all-trades athlete and have the ability to quickly analyze and appreciate the movement requirements for different sports, which come in handy when clients walk in the door with an interesting but obscure sport's injury. I have had the opportunity to work with many different athletes, but three groups in particular stand out in my mind as interesting learning experiences: the pole dancers from Tantra Fitness; a salesman-turned-professional fighter; and the Cirque du Soleil Delirium performers.

As it turns out, "pole fitness" is a sport that is growing in popularity all around the world, and I may now be one of the most experienced physiotherapists at working with these dancers, thanks to my client, Janet, the 2014 pole fitness champion. I started working with her in 2013, when she was balancing her work, as a speech language pathologist (SLP) at the nearby children's hospital, with numerous international pole fitness competitions. She was an ex-gymnast and had the perfect combination of bendiness and strength to excel at this new sport, and I had to quickly learn to think upside down and sideways to keep up with the demands she was putting on her body.

She trained hard, and as a life-long athlete she understood that she needed an equal amount of maintenance work to help keep her at her best and to prevent an injury from slowing her down. She came in regularly to my clinic for massage and physiotherapy appointments and realized the value of IMS (intramuscular stimulation) treatments for her pain, strength and flexibility; and she shared her secret with at least fifteen of her fellow athletes at Tantra. I started seeing two to three pole dancers a day for a while, all who were gluttons for punishment and hoping that IMS could give them the flexibility they needed to improve their next performance, and most of the time it did.

After seeing Janet through a variety of national and international competitions, I was given the opportunity to see her through an even bigger challenge—pregnancy. I watched her transition from a tiny, muscular dancer, to a very pregnant SLP, to a new mom, and back to a dancer again in the span of a few years. I can think of few sports that require more abdominal strength than pole dancing, and no life event compromises a person's core strength more than pregnancy with a C-section delivery and a diastasis of the linea alba (a split down the center of the six-pack muscles), but Janet wanted to return to the pole, so that was our goal. Her abdominals had been stretched to the point of tearing vertically and were then surgically cut horizontally, but the combination of her persistence, my guidance, and the capacity of the human body to heal got her back onto the pole in under a year's time.

Working with Janet helped reinforce my philosophy of release, re-educate, rebuild. I used IMS to loosen her clenching hip and back muscles, while keeping her aware of her posture and how pregnancy had affected it. I monitored the separation in her abdominals and referred her to clinical Pilates to retrain her deep core, and then helped to progressively layer on higher-level strengthening exercises until I felt she was safe to try the pole again. Once she returned, her knowledge of how to get stronger exceeded mine, so I dropped my role back to being her maintenance guy and watched her get stronger and stronger until she was upside down again. It was a fun case to be a part of, and I am proud of how well she has done.

Another sport that has exploded in the past decade has been mixed martial arts (MMA). I found myself in the middle of it for a while with a client, Carl, who was a salesman by day and a professional fighter by night. I even went out to the casino one night to watch what I was helping facilitate, because his fight was the main event and I wanted to see his world firsthand; it was slightly different from that of the pole dancers. Carl's world involved a combination of kick-boxing, wrestling, and intricate submission holds that required a whole different type of power, strength and toughness. He was a stand-up fighter with plenty of showmanship that crowds of tattooed musclemen ate up, but, unfortunately, he wasn't tougher than the herniated disc in his neck.

Working with competitive athletes comes with an entirely different set of goals than working with an average client. You have to strike a balance of working toward what is best for the person's body and what is best for their next performance, and sometimes the two goals don't line up. Athletes are more than willing to sacrifice their bodies for their sport, but sometimes a healthcare professional must help them know where to draw the line for the sake of their future, both personally and athletically. I had to be that person for Carl. He didn't have a lot of money and was bouncing back and forth between myself, a chiropractor, and a few massage therapists to keep him going. He was battling neck pain and shoulder weakness, but his symptoms were deceiving, because he had a very high pain threshold and was incredibly strong to start. He was having trouble finishing guys in submission holds, because he seemed to be losing the necessary arm power.

He was a difficult guy to rein in, because he kept bouncing around to different practitioners in search of temporary relief; that was, until I spent the time to explain that he had a significant disc herniation in his neck which was responsible for both his pain and his weakness. I told him that he would probably need to take an entire year away from fighting—and possibly have surgery—if he wanted to get back to 100%, and that if he continued on his current path, both his performance and his health would be seriously compromised. It took some effort, but I got through to him and helped him get better by doing less instead of more. He focused on work, underwent surgery and returned to competition a year later, better and stronger than ever, because he pulled the shoot and stopped when he needed to.

The group that had a hybrid of Carl and Janet's issues was the Cirque du Soleil performers who I had the opportunity to work with backstage during their local tour. They typically had a physiotherapist who traveled with them, but she was taking a course, so I filled her shoes for a few days and had fun doing it. The Delirium show had a combination of acrobats, gymnasts, and musicians who had been on the road for months traveling across North America and performing one or two shows a day. The performers, who were from all over the world, popped in and out of the medical room in various degrees of costume for a few hours before the show began. There were guys walking by on stilts, clowns pre-makeup, dancing and singing. I was literally backstage at a circus. Twelve performers at each show would sign up for a fifteen-minute physiotherapy slot, and I had to assess and help them so they could get out there to work their magic on stage a few hours later.

It was a mill of finely-tuned athletes who were all putting the show ahead of their pain. Some of them needed a manipulation, some a massage, and some just a new person to talk to because they had been on the road for so long with the same people. One short, muscular Russian gymnast came in, did a one-armed handstand, and said that his back hurt when he did this. Since I couldn't say, "Uh . . . don't do that," we had to problem solve quickly and work on his ribs. I didn't actually see the show until I had worked with them for a few days, but all their aches and pains made much more sense after I saw what they were doing, day in and day out. The time for rest and healing was after the tour, and our job was to patch them up as best we could because the show must go on! The experience taught me a great deal about priorities and being up front with what people want from you, while challenging them on what they truly need.

Although I enjoy working with high-level athletes, the experience always reminds me that I prefer the problem-solving aspect of trying to help people fix their resistant or chronic pain issues. I will always embrace sports and athleticism, but I find that seeing clients across a broad spectrum of abilities makes me better at dealing with all my clients, because I have a clearer perspective on what the body can do, for the better and for the worse. It's beneficial to see the ex-pro athletes who can barely walk, the aging weekend warriors, the average teenage soccer players, and the eighty-five-year-old grandmothers in the same day. You better know your place in life when you are regularly exposed to where you've been and where you might go, which is why I believe we need to connect kids with elite athletes and elite athletes with retired ones.

Now in my mid-thirties, with one good eye and a wonky shoulder to show for my athletic lifestyle, I am struggling to determine where sports fit into my life. I've gone through the being-patched-up-to-play phase, the fit-and-healthy phase, the forced-rest-phase, and now am wading into what looks like a transition to coaching stage. Some people don't understand why athletes punish themselves for the sports they love, but I'm sure most athletes would tell you it's just part of who they are and they wouldn't have it any other way. From a health perspective, sports and exercise in moderation are much better for you than not playing at all, but some of us need to take the "go big or go home" approach to life to be who we are, and we live with the consequences.

# What Is Your Core?
# It Depends On Who You Ask

The word "core" has been popular for quite a while now in the health, fitness, and rehab worlds, but there is no true agreement as to what it actually means; it depends on who you talk to. If you ask physiotherapists, most will focus on the deep, subtle, picky muscles like your transverse abdominus. If you ask strength and conditioning coaches, most will strive to build bracing stability using the obliques. If you ask Pilates instructors, most will focus on breathing and dissociation of movement. Finally, if you ask a layperson, most will just pat their stomach and say, "I know I need to work on my core," without really knowing why.

So who's right and who's wrong? The answer is, you should be able to selectively use your body for whatever task you ask it to do. The picky little muscles should work subconsciously while you stand, sit, walk, and breathe. The bracing muscles should work when you pick up or push something heavy, and you should be able to bend, twist, and stretch if you choose. The people who are wrong are the ones who believe their method is the only and best approach for everyone. Typically, personal trainers need to be introduced to Pilates instructors, and Pilates instructors require some personal training of their own. Most people have a need to work on something, but it is a misconception that building more strength and stability is always the best option.

Some people are naturally strong and stiff as a board, while others are loose-jointed with low muscle tone. The first and best thing you can do for yourself before you attempt more of anything physically is to learn about your body type, and what type of exercise would provide the greatest benefit to you. You may think yoga will make you looser, or that weight training will make you stronger, but they may also make you too tight or sore.

The first thing to understand about your muscles is that they are all in a big tug-of-war with each other. Some muscles are built to work together, while others pull against each other; when overly contracting, some muscle groups can and will inhibit other muscles from working properly. The best way to correct your posture and build core control is to learn what muscles you are overusing and try to figure out how to tone them down. It is more difficult to learn how to stop doing something you have done for years than it is to learn something new, but this is how strength becomes a skill. You need to learn how to efficiently harness the strength that you have by coordinating the muscles that are supposed to work together, while dampening down the ones that are trying to do everything. You can work for years to strengthen a specific muscle, but you won't grow stronger until you learn how to functionally use it with the rest of your body.

Your abdominals (abs) are a prime example. Everybody has an upper and lower body, but most people have trouble making them cooperate with each other; this is where your abs play an important role. To generalize, your back muscles work together with your thigh muscles, and your abdominals work with your butt and hamstrings. Most people find it easy to use their back and thighs but have trouble mastering the skill of recruiting their abs and glutes together, so the tendency is to get strong and tight in their back and thighs and weak and inhibited in their glutes and abs. Your abs connect the front of your rib cage to the front of your pelvis, while your back muscles do the opposite; they will lift your chest up and tip your torso backward. Unfortunately, this is the strategy most people will use to try and stand up straight with what they feel is "good posture." The result only makes them lean backward and inhibits the abs and glutes while compressing the lower back. The goal of posture and proper spine loading is to vertically elongate the spine and stack it in a neutral position, so as to not lift the chest up as much as possible. Movements that overly pull the lower ribs up and away from the front of the pelvis stretch and inhibit the abdominals from working properly.

The missing link to most people's idea of correct posture and core control is the internal support that the diaphragm plays in stabilizing the torso. Your diaphragm is comprised of the two big half-domes that sit inside the lower part of your rib cage and help you to breathe. It also helps support the weight of your torso off of your lower back and assists in preventing you from tipping backward when you stand up straight. Think of it as a mediator between the tug-of-war that is happening between your back muscles and your abs: the diaphragm helps put your trunk in a position so that your abs can stabilize the trunk. When it is not working well, the tendency is to overuse the back muscles to stabilize, which leads to stiffness and compression in the spine.

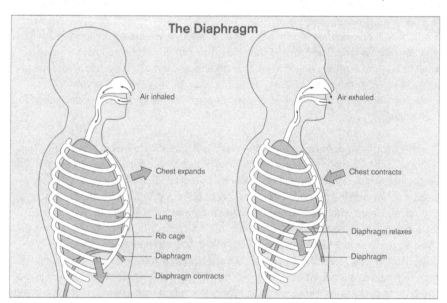

The diaphragm is comprised of two big muscular domes inside your lower trunk. Imagine opening a small umbrella inside your rib cage.

Our bodies are primarily built to deal with gravity in the vertically erect position. When an imbalance starts to develop in your gut-and-butt and back-and-thighs pairings, your torso will start to lean backward; where exactly it leans from will depend on the rest of your joints, but inevitably people develop a head-forward posture and will overly brace with their shoulders, butt, or thighs. I believe that if it took you A, B, and C to get where you are today, then you should trace your path back through C, B, and A to figure out how to perform it all properly. In other words, learn where you are bracing and try to stop it, and then try to figure out how to achieve a vertically stacked position, followed by trying to use muscles in that position. You will find that if you discover how to vertically stack everything, the picky, deep stabilizing muscles that physiotherapists teach you may switch on by themselves, and you will realize that there are a number of muscles in your body that you weren't using before. This is why it is important to spend most of your time training your core when you are on your feet and vertical, not horizontal on the floor.

Sometimes people are so subconsciously committed to their current posture and movement patterns that trying to change them is too overwhelming and seems impossible; this is when lying down to try and isolate muscle groups and working on dissociation of movement and breathing is important. The people who need this most are usually the "Type A" personalities who grip and brace everything. They would most benefit from yoga and Pilates, but would probably hate doing it and instead opt for a personal trainer to whip them into shape. The mellow, body-attuned people with dance backgrounds love lying on the floor and doing stretchy, bending exercises and may hate the whole gym scene, but they also need to branch away from Pilates and learn how to develop strength and power to lift, push, and pull.

The essence of developing core strength and stability is learning how to coordinate your upper and lower body to work together in a way that promotes strength, balance, and free movement. Some people may need to begin with physiotherapy, some with Pilates, and others in a gym program, but the fundamentals of movement are the same for everyone: you have to figure out what works best for you.

**Myth: If you have lower back pain, that means your "core is weak" and a "core strengthening" program would help you.**

Sometimes the above statement is true, but just as often it is completely false. There is no direct correlation between lower-back pain and core strength. In fact, many people with incredibly strong "core" muscles suffer from regular lower-back pain, because strength is only one element of good posture, alignment, and movement. It is the overall muscle balance in your body and your relative ability to control movement that is the true sign of good core stability and a preventative factor to lower-back pain.

Many people are stiff as a boards, and often these people suffer lower back pain and believe their planks, crunches, and strength programs will make them better. Well, I am here to tell you that there is a good chance it will make them worse. Granted, some will get better, but the most efficient way to improve your strength, flexibility, alignment, and pain is to first learn about your body type before pursuing a new program.

As you learned to function in the vertical position from a very young age, you developed strategies for how your body dealt with gravity. You picked up habits by watching how your parents stood, walked, and moved. You picked up other habits from your gymnastics classes and soccer practices when you were six. The hard fall you suffered on your butt twenty years ago likely had an impact, and that car accident five years ago probably created compensations. Essentially, your posture, flexibility, movement, and breathing patterns are a reflection of your past and present self.

You have ingrained movement patterns for how you balance and stabilize, which typically result in one type or another of imbalance and form a variety of bracing strategies. Instead of using your entire body equally to move and balance, you immediately migrate to what you know. Some people subconsciously brace their butt to hold themselves up, others brace their mid back, and still others their chest. Some people brace everything. When you encourage someone who uses a variety of bracing strategies to do more, you will likely feed their imbalances. The trouble is that the person will likely see good results initially, because they will become physically stronger, but quite often they will hit a plateau and/or start developing pain and injuries.

The best core program for bracers and grippers is one that focuses on movement awareness and working to correct everything that the person is bad at. It is much more difficult to unlearn a movement strategy than it is to learn a new one. People who are accustomed to using rigidity as their stabilizing strategy need to be introduced to mobility, and once they can learn to let go of their bracing, starting a strengthening program is appropriate. One-on-one Pilates, Feldenkrais training, and some types of yoga are good examples of movement leading to strength.

I was first introduced to the term "butt gripper" when I worked with Diane Lee and discovered that I, in fact, was one. As I became more body aware, I realized just how much I actually clenched my butt when I was standing—it blew me away. The more I assertively attempted to not clench, the better my back and hips started to feel.

In summary, some people can very much benefit from pure core strengthening programs, but others should stay away. It's best to learn about your body type and posture first, then learn to build targeted strength and practice movements that require improvement. Try not to stick to your favorite exercises that you are good at, because you will most likely only feed your imbalances.

## The Deep Inner Unit

Your deep inner unit consists of four muscle groups that should work subconsciously to stabilize your pelvis, spine, and rib cage under low-load postures and movements like standing, bending, and walking. Accidents, injuries, pregnancy, and developed muscle imbalances can cause portions of the deep inner unit to not properly do their job. The result can be pain and/or compensation from other muscle groups in trying to brace when holding everything together. Some of your other stronger muscles, such as your glutes, can make up for the deep inner unit, but this often leads to too much compression on the joints and immobility in the area. You function best when your body can use the little muscles for light activities and the bigger muscles for the more complex ones. You can get away with purely building strength in your outer sling muscles, but you will be prone to breaking down more often if the little muscles aren't firing.

The four muscle groups are your pelvic floor, transverse abdominus, multifidus, and diaphragm. They form the bottom, front, back, and top of your abdominal and pelvic cavity. Recruitment of these muscles is more about thinking than doing. They provide gentle compression to stabilize your pelvis and torso so that your bigger muscles can move your body. Although becoming aware of these muscles and consciously training them can be very important, they are supposed

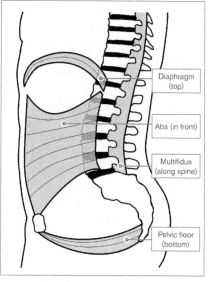

The four muscle groups that form the bottom, front, back and top of your abdominal and pelvic cavity.

to act subconsciously, and if you align your body in the proper way, they will likely fire on their own. I find it is the compensation strategies people choose in their posture that are inhibiting these deep inner unit muscles, and that helping a person unlearn their bracing strategies helps to fire up the deep inner unit more than trying to focus on them alone. This unit is an important entity that should not be overlooked, but it should also not be overly fixated on when it comes to dealing with back and pelvic pain.

Begin by objectively looking at your body type and your personality, and then asking yourself what is your physical goal before you start "working on your core." Consider both what you want to do and what you need to do before you pick your path, and don't be afraid to ask for guidance from a physiotherapist before you start. A focus on instilling good movement patterns before jumping into strengthening will always get you farther in the long run.

# Exercising for Your Body and Personality Type

We all come in different shapes and sizes, armed with our own personalities, but, unfortunately, we don't come with individualized instructional manuals on how to not wreck what we've been given. We have to figure it out on our own. The genetic lottery makes this task much easier for some than others, but all you need to worry about is your own body and not the annoyingly fit, strong, bendy person beside you. Life is not fair, so you need to work with what you're given and make the most out of it, or you will be forever unhappy with yourself.

The trouble is that body types and personality types don't always match up, so finding the best form of exercise to both appease the mind and not destroy the body can be tricky. I once treated a man in his mid-fifties who woke up in a hospital bed after suffering a heart attack and triple bypass surgery. He decided right then and there that he was going to do an Ironman race the next year, having never before competed in a triathlon. I met him four years and four Ironmans later as a short, thick, compressed man whose body needed a rest. His incredible determination got him into great shape, but it was also beating up on his joints to the point that they would stop him well before his heart or his brain would. I treated his pain and kept him going long enough to allow me to convince him to take a year off. A year of swimming and yoga helped his competition times more than a year of the intense personal training, running, and biking that he was doing, and he returned to the sport the next year in better comfort and with more enjoyment.

Having a goal is a major factor to getting what you want out of exercise, but many people don't know what exactly they want and believe they should exercise to be healthier. It's a good premise, but what it means to be healthier is closely related to who you are and where you are at, physically and emotionally. Exercise is healthy for the body and mind if you pick the right type, but one can come at the expense of the other if you don't consider why you are doing what you are doing. Your brain may need you to run five miles to put it at ease, but your back may prefer the swimming pool. Your body may feel as though it needs to stretch, but your mind may hate everything about yoga. Sometimes your body wants more and your mind wants less, and other times this is reversed. The ability to check in with yourself and determine what you need both mentally and physically is an important skill to develop.

I had played sports my entire life until I turned thirty-two, when we had our third child in three years and I just couldn't find the time to work, parent, and commit to a team, so I stopped playing soccer. It became the busiest yet most relatively sedentary period of my life in terms of traditional exercise, and it opened my eyes to what sports actually meant to me and did for me. I craved the competition, the physical challenges, and the camaraderie more than I needed the exercise. I have always been a tall, lean person who couldn't gain weight if I tried, so sports and exercise, I learned, were more a requirement of my mind than my body. I went stir crazy without sports and began looking for ones that I could fit into my tightly packed schedule.

I started playing squash twice a week with friends who were less athletic than me but who were better squash players, and I had to endure a year of losing before I started to level the playing field. It got me out of the house, gave me the competition I needed, and made me sweat for an hour; my mind and body were happy. I had to realize that exercise couldn't just spontaneously happen for me anymore: it needed to be in my schedule. I tried running occasionally but found my body became sore and my brain grew bored. I went to the gym a few times but realized that I'd spent enough time in my life in a gym and didn't enjoy being there, so I stopped. Exercise should be enjoyable, so I found a group of guys who played ball hockey once a week, and I was set. My brain and body had just settled into the pattern of squash and hockey once a week when my world got flipped upside down with my eye injury, and I went back to being more sedentary than before.

When I started Envision Physiotherapy in 2006, it was just me in a room in the corner of a fitness center trying to make my presence known. I offered countless free assessments to new gym members to start building my caseload, and met many lost souls who were joining the gym because they thought they should, not because they wanted to. It was that experience that led me to dissuade many people from "working out" and instead encouraged them to explore other physical activities like hiking, swimming, dancing, Pilates, yoga, and various sports. Some people are meant for the gym and others should avoid it unless they are able to do it one-on-one with a personal trainer. I believe any new physical undertaking should begin with some basic instruction on skill development and appropriate frequency because many people, left to their own devices, end up hurting themselves.

Your body type should be an important factor when considering what exercise you choose and what your expectations should be. The first factor is where you fall on a scale of hypermobility (see Section 1, "Getting Old Sucks"). The second is your physical stature: are you tall and lean, or short and stout? Finally, how do you think your underlying posture and alignment will affect your activity of choice? Your mind may want to do something, but sometimes you should consider whether your body is up for the task, as well as whether you are prepared to undertake the necessary maintenance to keep going. Some people are built to do triathlons and some aren't, but I see all shapes and sizes out there trying!

Hypermobile people who get into Olympic lifting often run into trouble. Stocky, hypomobile people who try to run marathons end up in physiotherapy before they reach the finish line. Stiff, competitive people who attempt yoga hurt their backs when trying to get more flexible. People with rounded upper backs run into neck trouble when they cycle long distances. Scoliosis and alignment problems can make both staying still and carrying heavy loads problematic. There are endless combinations that you could say, "Yeah, of course you got hurt," to, ut the human spirit usually trumps logic and awareness. We want to do the activities that we enjoy, and that is fine—it is part of what gives me a job as a physiotherapist—but I emphasize my point: ask yourself why you want to do something before you start. If your goal is to stay fit and healthy and to not hurt yourself, then consider your body's capacity before your mind's. If you love a sport and will do anything to compete and succeed despite the impact on your body, then have a team of health professionals around you to better know the problems to watch out for and when to put on the brakes.

A good physiotherapist should be able to teach you about your own body and give you guidelines to exercising without hurting yourself, but it is up to you to actually practice what you have learned. Health is a relative issue, and everyone has the capacity to both improve and erode; it takes conscious effort to improve, but only ignorance or neglect to erode. If you are having any doubts about your body and want to stay fit while exercising, I recommend checking in with a physiotherapist every four to six weeks for a tune-up and feedback on how and what you are doing.

# Yoga and Stretching Injuries: Why People Get Injured on Their Quest for Bendiness

It seems like everyone these days is either doing yoga or feels that they should be for some reason. Its popularity has steadily grown over the past ten years to include a more and more diverse group of people. Businessmen, athletes, seniors, and children have all joined in the sun salutations and downward dogs in a quest for flexibility and inner peace. For the most part, I think this movement is great, but as a physiotherapist I see countless injuries, postural issues, and persistent pains that have their roots in people's regular yoga routines. There are many benefits to yoga, but it is not meant for everyone, and you can have too much of a good thing. This article discusses some of those negative consequences of yoga—not to scare you away from it, but to help you go into yoga armed with the awareness of how not to hurt yourself.

Before you decide to start any new type of exercise, you should ask yourself, "What am I trying to get out of this?" Many people blindly feel that yoga is the answer to flexibility, and although it can be for some, it can also be an awkward, uncomfortable path to injury for others. Flexibility is partly genetic but largely a product of what you do all day: how you stand, sit, walk, breathe, and feel affect your flexibility. It is a misconception that you are stiff because you don't spend enough time stretching. You are stiff because you either don't move enough or you don't move very well, or both. Stretching more is simply not the answer. In fact, there are millions of hours wasted every day by people stretching in attempt to become more flexible. Some people will gain benefit, some won't, and some will actually end up tighter from trying to stretch; which one will you be?

Yoga can be a calming stress reliever for some people, and they are the ones who typically gain the most benefit. Finding a mind-body connection that relates to movement is essential to create change in your body. Simply going through the motions and forcing yourself into specific poses won't get you very far and can initiate a tug-of-war with your body that you are likely to lose. In order to do stretching-based exercises effectively, it is important to understand where the tightness that you feel in your body is originating. Not all tight feelings should be stretched, and a feeling of tightness does not necessarily mean that you should try to increase your flexibility of that area.

The structure of your body is a bony framework that is held together by muscles, tendons, ligaments, and connective tissue called fascia. There is a genetic variability from person to person in how tightly all these tissues hold you together. Some people are genetically loose-jointed or hypermobile, while others are tightly packed together or hypomobile. As imagined, the hypermobile people are naturally more flexible than their counterparts, but what you wouldn't expect is that they typically feel the stiffest.

Hypermobile people have great flexibility but typically feel stiff, as though they should be stretching, and tend to take pleasure from activities like yoga. Hypomobile people, meanwhile, tend to have awful flexibility and feel guilty when they don't stretch enough; they don't necessarily feel tight, but stretching doesn't often help the problem and doesn't feel good, so they don't bother.

We function in the vertical or erect position. We spend long periods of time standing, sitting, walking, pushing, pulling, lifting or bending, all with gravity trying to drag us down. Some of us are tightly held together and others loosely, but we all have the same basic anatomy and the same challenge of trying to keep our bodies vertical throughout the day. No one teaches you how to stack up everything when you are young, but everyone figures out their own way to move based on their genetics, sports, injuries, and personalities. Starting from a very young age, children develop muscle imbalances and inefficient movement patterns that can mold how they stand, sit and walk for the rest of their lives. As an adult, you take most of these basic movement patterns for granted, but as I have said before, just because you can stand, sit, and walk does not mean that you do it very well.

Below is an illustration taken from my article "Why Hips Hurt: An Illustrated Explanation." It shows examples of common postures and muscle imbalances that develop in people over time. Each imbalance creates its own kinks and hinges in the spine, both as you move and as you attempt to stay still. Some vertebrae or joints

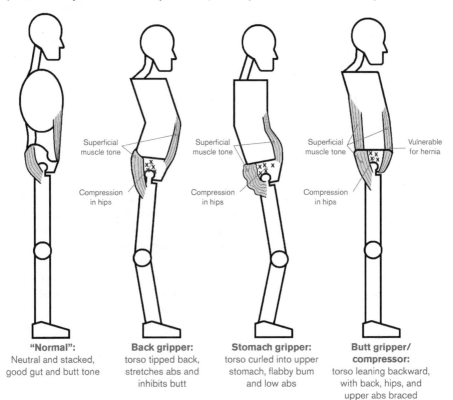

**"Normal":**
Neutral and stacked, good gut and butt tone

**Back gripper:**
torso tipped back, stretches abs and inhibits butt

**Stomach gripper:**
torso curled into upper stomach, flabby bum and low abs

**Butt gripper/ compressor:**
torso leaning backward, with back, hips, and upper abs braced

become overly compressed and others are over-stretched. Typically, when one area doesn't move enough, somewhere else will move too much, and vice-versa.

When you are vertical, your spine and the nerves that extend from it are happiest when you stay in more or less a "neutral" position. Neutral refers to the natural S-curve in your spine. This is not to imply that you should never move out of this neutral position, but you should become aware of how easy or difficult this position is for you to attain. Ideally, you can move through your entire spine in a controlled manner or stabilize it back into this neutral S-curve. You should also be able to coordinate and control the movement of your lower body and your trunk, but unfortunately, due to some of the above common postural imbalances, this can become a challenge.

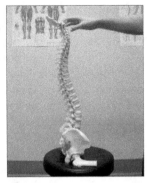

Neutral, or natural S-curve of the spine.

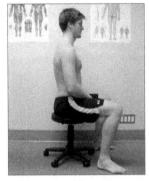

Proper sitting position allowing for neutral position of the spine.

Poor movement and postural patterns will, over time, lightly annoy various nerve roots as they extend from your spine. These nerve roots are like the electrical wiring extending from a fuse box to all the muscles, joints, and organs throughout your body. When nerves become annoyed, they get overly sensitive and can start creating bands of tension in your muscles; this tension will affect your flexibility and may give you the sensation that you want to stretch that muscle. The trouble is that the muscle is not only shortened and needing to be stretched, it is that a portion of it is lightly contracting all the time, even at rest, because the nerve that innervates it is annoyed. Trying to stretch that type of muscle can be counterproductive and may lead to injury; this happens in yoga often.

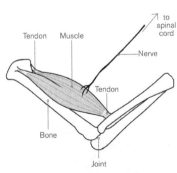

**Normal state muscle**

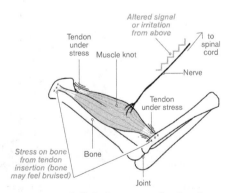

**Irritated nerve causing tension**

You need to teach your body how to make the muscle stop contracting, and not continue stretching it. Intramuscular stimulation (IMS) is the quickest and most effective way to reset this negative muscle tone, but various myofascial release techniques like lying on a tennis ball and consciously trying to relax a trigger point can be helpful too. What you need to learn going into yoga is what a good stretch versus a bad stretch might feel like. When you move into a stretch position your muscles, nerves, joints and fascia will all dictate how much you move. A good stretch should not be forced; it should be gentle and feel like a nice lengthening feeling through the middle of the muscle. If you end up trying to stretch muscles that are full of taut bands due to nerve irritation, it can feel like a stronger stretch sensation at the ends of muscles, more in the tendons and joints. This is something to be wary of, as successful stretching is not a "more pain, more gain" exercise. Unfortunately, when you put a large group of people with various body types into a yoga class, the competitive nature of people can be revealed, and injuries can be the result.

Movement follows the law of physics: your joints will take the path of least resistance as you move. For example, if you are a back gripper, you likely have a tight back that doesn't flex very well but have very flexible hamstrings, so when you bend forward, you tend to move mostly in your hips and not your back.

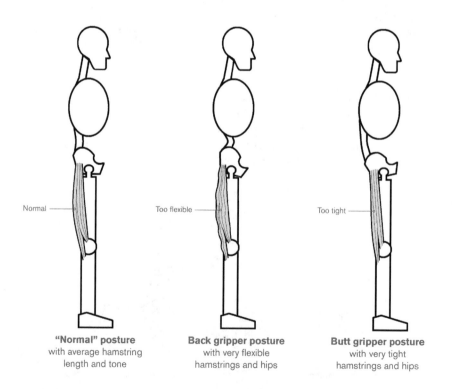

| "Normal" posture | Back gripper posture | Butt gripper posture |
| --- | --- | --- |
| with average hamstring length and tone | with very flexible hamstrings and hips | with very tight hamstrings and hips |

Conversely, if you are a butt gripper, you would tend to have tight hips and hamstrings, and forward bending would happen mainly from your back (see below). These differences in people can lead to varying results when you ask a room of thirty people to all hold the same poses.

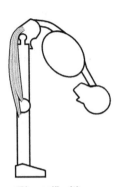 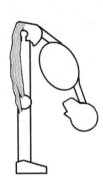 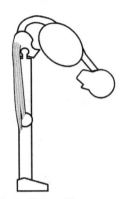

| **"Normal" with average hamstrings:** | **Back gripper with long hamstrings:** | **Butt gripper with tight hamstrings:** |
|---|---|---|
| bends partly in hips and partly in spine | flexes mostly in hips; hamstrings don't control the movement well | flexes mostly in spine; hamstrings don't permit much hip movement |

You might be surprised to learn which group comprises the majority of yoga injuries. In my experience, it is 20% of the stiff guys who push it too hard and 80% of the most hypermobile women who have done yoga for a long time. The most common yoga injury I see is hip and upper hamstring pain in women with overly flexible hips. When the glutes and hamstrings become too flexible bending forward, they aren't strong enough to functionally help the person with activities that require power in more normal ranges like standing, walking, or running. As a result, the person's back and thigh muscles do most of the work and inevitably grow tight. Your back and thighs are then inefficient at helping you walk and run; it is your butt and hamstrings that are supposed to push you forward. Over-flexibility in the back of the legs and the resulting muscle imbalances tends to create tension in the deep stabilizing muscles of the hips, like the piriformis. Too much tension in these muscles will annoy the sciatic nerve and create a feeling of tightness in the hamstring and hip; this is the trap that many "yogies" fall into. That tight feeling in the upper hamstring is just begging to be stretched, but too much length in the muscle and relative weakness is how the problem originated. These people need to stop overly stretching their hips and hamstrings, and start working on trunk control and proper posture.

Many yoga exercises focus on whole-back extension and preach chest up, shoulders back and down. It complements the posture that most dancers develop over time, which is one reason dancers tend to migrate to yoga. As a physiotherapist, my experience is that although a dancer's posture can look esthetically nice, it is also responsible for a great deal of pain and dysfunction over time, and that laypeople

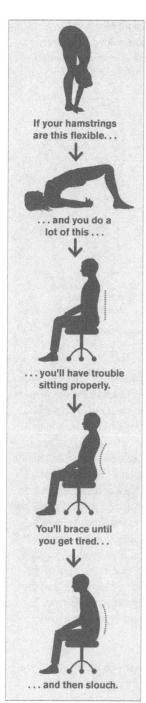

If your hamstrings
are this flexible...

↓

...and you do a
lot of this...

↓

...you'll have trouble
sitting properly.

↓

You'll brace until
you get tired...

↓

...and then slouch.

⬆ An overly flexible body can
cause problems when you
are sitting for long periods.

should not strive to look like dancers. Dancers' posture and mobility is great if you are going to be a dancer but awful if you have a desk job, want to be a runner, or do physical work. Some of the poses and cueing can lead to overuse of the back and shoulder muscles and generally poor awareness of how to stack up your spine in a strong position.

The basic cat/cow movement is an example; this is a good, general-mobility exercise for the spine and is easy for most people to perform. Most people need to learn that their trunk and pelvis can move independently of each other to make the spine look more like a snake than a cat or a cow.

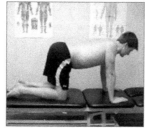
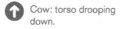
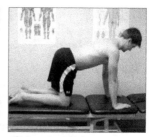

⬆ Cow: torso drooping
down.

⬆ Neutral spine: torso
supported.

The bridge is another example. Most yoga and Pilates cueing will have people lifting their rib cage and arching up their backs as much as possible; this practice disengages the butt and abs from working properly and exaggerates the back and shoulders of which many yogies are already too dominant. Most people need to learn how to use their gut and butt together in a more neutral position.

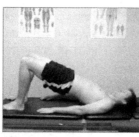
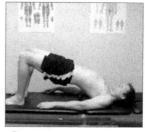

⬆ Bridge using gut and butt
together.

⬆ Bridge overusing back
instead of abs and butt.

Yoga poses tend to allow your body to move and take the plane of least resistance, which means you will move in the way that you are good at; this can be good to an extent, but too much can further develop your movement and postural problems. Challenging yourself to move in ways that you are bad at is the only method for creating functional change in your body; it is more mentally and physically challenging but also more productive.

That said, not all exercise needs to be productive. Moving for the sake of moving is sometimes all a person needs, but if you are doing yoga with the goal of improving your posture and flexibility, make sure you go into it with awareness of your body, and understand that all cues might not be right for you. Learn the fundamentals of your posture and movement, and consider these principles while you perform any type of exercise.

You may find the video progressions on WhyThingsHurt.com playlists will help you develop the building blocks of good posture and movement in preventing injury while you exercise. They are modifications of common exercises, taking into account the common muscle imbalances and what to watch out for.

Your muscle and postural imbalances, combined with your level of hyper/hypomobility, will very much affect your experience when you decide to take up yoga. I recommend learning to exercise for your body type and again ask yourself, "What am I trying to get out of this?" Is it flexibility, stress release, strength, pain relief, or rehabilitation? When you determine what you want, do your homework and find the right type of yoga for you; there are many different kinds. I would also consider the idea that maybe yoga isn't the right choice for you. Pilates or a good personal trainer might help you to build more functional strength and solve more of your problems. I would also consider consulting an experienced physiotherapist to help guide you in the right direction, or watch the videos on WhyThingsHurt.com to help improve your body awareness and basic movement patterns.

# Golfers: A Breed All Their Own

Early in my career, I spent two years working almost exclusively with golfers in Vancouver and a nearby suburb called White Rock as part of a small business that held the franchise rights to an American company called Body Balance for Performance. I was trained by the physiotherapist owner of the local company and then sent to Philadelphia for a week of training with the parent company. I learned about the principles of golf movement, how to speak golf lingo, and how to sell expensive, golf-centered fitness and treatment programs to aging wealthy golfers. In hindsight, it was a valuable experience that molded how I approached physiotherapy going forward.

I found that the sales training made me a better teacher, educator, and physiotherapist, because it taught me how to talk about the body in a way that was meaningful to a person who didn't care about anatomy. I learned how to wrap important information around a sport that its players were passionate about to help them help themselves and write me a check for two thousand dollars at the same time.

I spent hours every spring and summer standing in an open tent with a folding massage table on the edge of golf tournament driving ranges, performing quick assessments and treatments on executives before the shotgun of their tournaments, in an attempt to find new clients. The golfers who were intrigued enough by their interaction with me would come in for a two-to-three-hour head-to-toe evaluation and video analysis of their swing. I would explain how restrictions in their lead-hip rotation could be causing their back pain, or more importantly, their slice. I would open their eyes to just how poor their trunk rotation was and show them how it affected their distance and likely their shoulder pain. In the video, I could show them why they were hitting the ball thin or fat all the time, all based on their physical limitations. I would then propose a two-to-six-month plan of visits to treat their pain, loosen them up, and develop an exercise regimen to improve their consistency and distance based on their goals. Golfers loved it, but it wasn't cheap.

When most of my young physiotherapist friends were seeing three to four patients with acute pain every hour, I was spending one to three hours each with aging businessmen, teaching them how to move properly. I started on a different path and never quite merged back to being a "normal" physiotherapist. Starting with the chronically stiff and stubborn guys changed my perspective on how to exercise, knowing what was helpful and what was harmful, as well as what was a giant waste of time. Since I had ample time with clients and didn't have to worry about the acuity of their pain, I could better understand what made them tick and could be more specific with what I thought could help them. I gained an appreciation for the interconnection of body type, personality, and pain, because golf is such a physical and mental game that can hurt you if not done properly.

Golf, more than any sport I can think of, becomes an obsession for people. When someone has the time and money to devote to golfing, it can become a major priority in their life and lifestyle. It is a sport that, with enough dedication, someone can get close to mastering but can never perfect, so there is always a carrot dangling in front to work on something. Merchandisers take full advantage of the fact that golfers are suckers for gizmos to help their game, and typically have the money to pay for them. It was my job to convince the golfers in front of me that the best tool they had to improve their game was their body and not a new driver. Improving their body took time, but a new driver only took money, so many times the driver won out, but I could be fairly convincing at changing their behavior eventually.

The accepted model of exercising and rehabilitation that most people have followed for years is that their body needs either to be stretched or strengthened in order to improve, but working with countless golfers has effectively disproved that theory for me. I worked with guys who had spent the past ten years religiously stretching the same areas and still couldn't touch their toes, and others who had hired personal trainers to make them stronger, only to lose distance and hurt their backs. The experience taught me that good movement patterns are the most important part of function, and that strength is a skill developed on top of that. People who move well have very little need to stretch and have an easy time getting stronger. Conversely, people who work hard at getting stronger but don't learn how to move well end up compressing their nervous system and have to stretch or foam roll more often. (Foam rolling is a self-myofascial release (SMR) technique used by athletes and physical therapists to inhibit overactive muscles).

Golf is a finesse sport, but being strong can be an asset, so I tried to strike a balance with many of my clients in discussing how much their gym routine was helping versus hindering them. To move efficiently in a golf swing, the trunk needs to dissociate from the lower body in the back swing and then connect back up and shift the dissociation to the lead hip for the follow through. Rotational movements are most important, but many of my clients were "working on their core" by strengthening all the muscles that resisted rotation in their bodies, making their backs stronger and tighter.

*The following is an outline of the fundamentals of golf movement. The exercises listed can be found on my website at WhyThingsHurt.com*

Movement is a skill, and skill is the key component to strength. If you learn to move well, you will build functional strength. If you spend time trying to grow stronger and ignore movement, you will likely become functionally weaker and be prone to hurting yourself.

Golf is a game about finely controlled movement and cognitive management—two concepts that elude and frustrate people their entire lives, which is why golf can be so addictive. How a person approaches a golf game reflects much about their personality and their physical body, and both factors tend to contribute to their consistency, power, form and ultimately the number on the scorecard after eighteen holes. It also has much to do with how sore they are during or after a round.

Rotation is the obvious movement pattern that golfers need to master, but it is only one of three movement planes that exist in the golf swing, and it is by far the most complex. It is a mistake to try and address rotation until you first learn how to move in the forward-back and side-to-side planes. I tell my clients that they need to earn the right to rotate by first learning to squat properly and load their legs well. You would be surprised just how poorly most people bend or squat down, but it is a key part of the address position in a golf swing.

### Step 1: Learn where your hips actually are

- "4-Point Neutral Spine" video
- "4-Point Rock-backs" video

In order for your trunk to rotate properly, the muscles in your back should be reasonably relaxed, because they need to lengthen as your body turns. The way most people bend or squat ends up creating far too much tension in their back and butt to allow them to freely rotate their trunk. You need to learn how to bend over slightly using your legs and abs while maintaining a neutral spine. Neutral means a gentle S-curve, and not trying to stay vertical.

### Step 2: The address position: learn to bend using your legs and NOT your back

- "Kneeling Squats" video
- "How to Stand" video
- "Standing Squats" video
- "Thirsty Birds" video
- "The Address Position" video

Once you can stand and bend more effectively, the goal is to create more awareness of leg loading. By that I mean how to stack your hip on your knee and your knee on your foot to support your body in a balanced manner as you move. This is where most swing flaws are created; men tend to compensate for a lack of hip flexibility with hip slides and reverse pivots, while women tend to lose power by not using their legs in the swing. Learning to move laterally in a slight squat will expose leg tightness or weakness and teach you how to use your feet, knees, and hips together. The lateral movement in the golf swing is minimal, but important. You need to learn how to create strong, stable leg loading in your back swing and free movement leg loading in your follow through.

### Step 3: Become aware of your foot, knee, hip connection

- "Foot as a Tripod" video
- "Speed Skater" video
- "Squat + Lateral Movement" video

Now that you can squat and load your legs, it is time to discover your trunk. The first step is to understand that your trunk and your shoulders are two separate entities. Your rotation movement should come from your trunk and not your arms. Most people are fantastic at cheating to make up for their physical restrictions. Tightness in your trunk typically results in too much hip or arm movement during the swing. Your ability to rotate has much to do with your general posture and how you breathe. Learn about how you hold yourself, then sit down and try to dissociate your trunk from your pelvis and your neck–it is harder than you may think.

### Step 4: Learn the role of posture, breathing and dissociation

- "Everything your mother taught you about posture is WRONG" video
- "Rib Shimmy" video
- "Breathing as an Exercise" video
- "Seated-Trunk Rotation" video

Standing up and putting it all together can be a lot of things to think about at first, but if you break it down into parts, the golf swing is a coordinated series of biomechanics that can be repeated. If you understand each component in your body, you will then understand your swing and the flaws that you just can't seem to improve. When the exercises get closer and closer to resembling a golf swing, it is important to not use a club or even your arms, but to rather think biomechanics and not golf, because if you use a club or your arms then the old, ingrained patterns will want to take over.

### Step 5: Putting it all together: trunk rotation, coil and the lead hip

- "The Address Position" video
- "Standing Rotation" video
- "Back Swing: Trunk Rotation and Leg Loading" video
- "Down Swing & Follow Through: Lead-hip Rotation and Weight Transfer" video

Once you can discover the biomechanics of your golf swing, it is time to start using your arms again and even put a club in your hands; be aware, however, that your old habits will be lurking. Your job now is to focus on the movement patterns described above and work on keeping your arms connected to your trunk as you rotate. Staying connected can be challenging due to physical restrictions in your body, specifically your lats, chest, trunk, and hips. Performing movement-control exercises and targeted stretching can make all of the golf movements that much easier. Stretching alone will do almost nothing for you, but if you work on improving the movement patterns and add stretching, you will start to see some changes.

**Step 6: Golf-specific exercises for posture and flexibility**

- "Passive Chest Stretch" video

- "4 Point Rock-backs" video

- "Reaching up 11" video

- "Lat Stretch" video

- "Air Bench Press" video

- "Standing Trunk Rotation" video

- "Standing Hip Rotation" video

You will find that a golf professional can teach you the technical aspects of the game, but you will be confined by what your body allows him to teach. If you spend some time learning about your general posture and how you sit, stand, breathe, and walk and how that affects your flexibility and your golf game, your golf pro will have more to work with when it comes time for lessons.

Core strengthening programs can be helpful tools to improve your game and your general fitness level, but remember that strength is a skill, and that attempting to add strength on top of poor movement patterns may only take you backward in the long run.

If pain and tightness continue to be limiting factors and you feel as though you have tried everything, consider trying IMS (intramuscular stimulation). It can work wonders with stiff hips and bodies that haven't moved well in years.

# Shoes: Good Support or Coffins for Your Feet?

We are born barefoot and are genetically built to stand, walk, and run with our feet interacting with the ground. Our feet are built to be both shock absorbers and rigid levers for us to use in pushing off. They have allowed human beings to navigate uneven ground, hard, flat planes and soft, spongy meadows for thousands of years. It is only recently that we started flattening out our world with concrete, and supporting and cushioning our feet with fancy shoes and orthotics. The feedback our bodies get from our feet is a crucial aspect of posture, balance, and movement development, but we tend to almost immediately cut that off by putting our children in stiff, cushy running shoes as soon as they can walk. As people grow up, the role of work, fashion, and sport dictate their footwear choices, and it usually comes at the cost of body awareness, foot strength, and balance. As a result, it is almost the norm for people's feet to slowly deform over time and develop bunions, hammer toes, fallen arches, and plantar fasciitis. Ultimately, footwear choices become less and less about fashion as we age and more about cushioning and supportive comfort. This path is a major source of balance and pain issues throughout life.

The mechanics of our feet are closely tied to those of our hips. Tightness or weakness in one will directly affect the other, which ultimately affects the entire body. There are three main arches to the foot, the main one being the medial longitudinal arch; this is the part that will pronate (flatten) or supinate (arch up/over). There is also a smaller lateral arch along the outside of the foot, but the most overlooked arch is called the transverse and is supposed to dome up the front part of the foot. This arch collapses in most feet primarily due to wearing shoes all the time, only walking on flat ground, and our tendency to walk overly erect. The muscles on the bottom of the feet become extremely weak, the muscles in the calf get overworked, and as a result the mechanical support and leverage provide by the foot is lost. Pain, bunions, hammer toes, and plantar fasciitis follow closely behind.

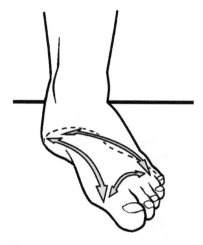

**Arches of the foot**

The foot is comprised of numerous small bones that require muscle tension along its length to hold them all together. When this muscle tension weakens, the bones cannot lock together effectively and the arches will collapse. The result is typically poor shock absorption for the body and poor load transfer of the work that is done by the rest of the leg. In other words, the hip and leg muscles work to extend your leg backward to propel you forward, but much of that energy is lost in the foot if it doesn't possess the strength to lock into a rigid lever to push off. This is an example of an inefficiency of movement, and when it happens with every step you take, the result is usually a tightening of the hip muscles and eventually pain in the foot, knee, or lower back.

When the mechanics of your feet are compromised, your glutes are not able to do their job properly. When your glutes aren't working well, your deep rotator muscles underneath them and your groin muscles are overworked in trying to stabilize your hip. These muscles play a key role in the alignment of your pelvis and the orientation of how your hips sit in their sockets. The deep muscles in the hip tend to rotate the leg outward, while the groin muscles tend to rotate the leg inward. How your leg functions depends on which muscles are winning this tug-of-war. Typically, if the hip muscles are winning, the leg rotates outward, your foot overly supinates and you put most of your weight on the outside of your foot; if your groin muscles are winning, the leg rotates inward, your foot overly pronates and you load too much weight on the inside of your foot. If your leg becomes bowed or knock-kneed, it can become even more complicated, but as you can see, there is a close relationship between your feet and your hips. There is a trickle-up and a trickle-down effect, and both are equally important.

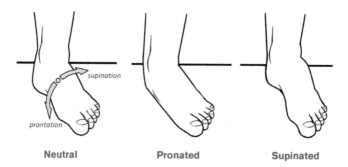

**Neutral**          **Pronated**          **Supinated**

Unfortunately, the accepted practice of dealing with foot issues is to try and solve everything by giving people stiffer and more supportive shoes and orthotics; this practice usually helps people who pronate and hinders people who supinate. The pronaters are happy with their motion-control shoes and orthotics, but they become reliant on them and run into trouble when sandal season comes around. The supinaters, meanwhile, want to believe their orthotics are helping them (because they cost $500) but they usually either make no difference or make the person even worse. Cushioning and support are good for your feet when you are in pain. When you are not in pain, however, giving your feet a chance to do some work and experience the ground is the best thing for them and the rest of your body.

It is not realistic to expect everyone to stop wearing shoes, but there are a growing number of flatter, more flexible shoes on the market that protect your feet while allowing them to work. Some women will always wear high heels, but if they don't want killer calves, ugly feet, and a painful back, they should consider switching occasionally to flats and take their shoes off as much as possible. It is easy to opt for the shoe that is the warmest and cushiest, but I warn you that what feels good in the short term may be harmful in the long run. The best compromise is to buy a variety of shoes and use the flat ones as training tools to strengthen your feet and to become aware of your posture.

The best thing that I ever did for my feet, my posture, and my foot pain was to stop wearing traditional shoes. I am hypermobile and have very high arches in my feet, which I now realize were the causes of the foot pain and blood blisters that slowed me down throughout my entire athletic life. I had tried all different types of shoes, orthotics, and tapes, so in 2008 I decided to start working in only socks most of the day, and I never turned back. Going shoeless taught me a great deal about my own body and how I was creating my own hip and back pain. The feedback I was receiving from my feet helped me to become aware that I was standing entirely on the outsides of my feet and how that related to the tightness and aching in my hips. From the ground up, I progressively became aware of how one part of my body was affecting the other, and I have been able to successfully strengthen my feet, loosen my hips and eliminate almost all of the chronic issues I was suffering.

Being a physical therapist and seeing fourteen people a day with different body and foot types has allowed me to test my posture and movement principles on myself as well as on my clients. I have helped many people discover how their feet affect their bodies and how their bodies affect their feet. I have learned that how you hold your upper body can be the root cause of your bunions, and that how you use your hips can dictate if you pronate or supinate in your feet. The shoes you choose will affect all of the above.

Let me walk you through the path I have taken to create strong feet and good posture as it relates to my shoes. The first fact to consider is that we are all born and built to function barefoot; you were not born with Nikes on. The second fact is that your body adapts to the forces you put on it; it will compensate and adapt to the shoes you have chosen throughout life, usually in a negative way. These compensations and adaptations happen over years and typically catch up to you sooner or later in the form of pain or deformity in your feet, knees, or back; your body is built to function one way, but you have forced it to function in another. If you truly want to restore normal functioning, it takes time, concentration, and persistence to undo the deeply-ingrained movement patterns and weaknesses in your feet and body.

I started by taping up my feet in a way that compensated for all my weaknesses; the tape performed the mechanical action my weak muscles weren't able to provide. The results were incredible. I felt twenty pounds lighter. My toes straightened out instead of bunching up, and I could feel my feet become levers to push me forward when I was walking. To top it all off, it got rid of my foot pain. I started taping up most of my clients' feet, and 75% of them found the same result. The trouble was that the tape job only lasted about two days, and it became impractical to tape all the time, but it motivated me to strengthen my feet and made me further realize how traditional shoes were causing my problems.

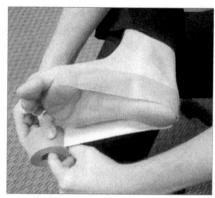

Search "Toe Spreader" on WhyThingsHurt.com for the video of this tape job.

The foot is built to bear weight on the heel, the lateral portion of the sole, the ball of the forefoot, and the toes–just what you would see in a footprint on the ground. The front of the foot is supposed to flex and extend like the ankle can. You should be able to wave goodbye with your forefoot, but shoes don't permit foot flexion, only extension. Your feet are built to grab the ground and lightly contour to the surface to help provide balance and support to the body, but shoes prevent your feet from doing any work by artificially lifting you away from the ground and providing a gripped, stable base. Shoes can make certain activities easier for your body, but they can be coffins for your feet. Imagine what would happen to your hands if you wore mittens all the time that didn't let you make a fist, grip, or use any dexterity. They would eventually deform and your fingers would curl up, just like most toes do in shoes.

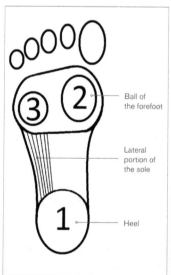

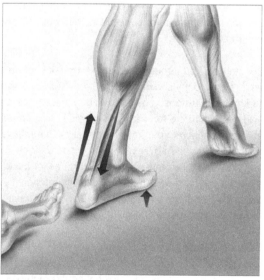

Foot should bear weight like a tripod and have lengthwise tension for support.

Feet are built to grab the ground and lightly contour to the surface for balance and support.

People have come to believe that they require the support that shoes and orthotics provide—and some truly do—but most people need the support because of the shoes they have been wearing their whole life, and not because they are meant to have something pushing their arch up from below. You can become dependent on your shoes and orthotics and can progressively require stiffer and more supportive shoes over time as your feet become weaker and weaker. This is the path many people choose, because it can demonstrate the most immediate comfort, but I warn that this can lead to balance and pain issues later in life. I encourage people to learn how to use their feet in conjunction with the rest of their body, to naturally build arches and strong feet; this process takes time but pays dividends in the long run. If you are older, and your feet have already developed large bunions and hammer toes, your best option may be to compensate for your feet with supportive shoes and orthotics, but most people could benefit from shedding their traditional shoes even part of the time and go for a barefoot walk.

The footwear industry has started to shift toward a minimalist mentality when it comes to athletic shoes. There are a handful of companies starting to produce their version of a "barefoot shoe." These are extremely light shoes that protect your feet from sharp objects but don't provide much cushioning or support; they let your feet do the work. Most traditional running shoes have an elevated, cushioned heel, a stiff midfoot section, and a relatively thinner sole in the forefoot. Compared to going barefoot, running shoes are high heels that promote heel striking and make it challenging to use the front of your foot properly.

Nike was the first major company to develop a more minimalist shoe with their Nike Free line. The Free is extremely light and has slats in the sole that allow more movement to occur in the foot, but it still has the elevated profile of a traditional running shoe. The heel is typically higher than the forefoot, and the shoe facilitates more extension in the forefoot, but still doesn't allow it to flex. I view this shoe as a good transition toward going barefoot.

Vibram developed their Five Fingers shoe around 2006, which seemed to start the barefoot movement. Their shoe is the closest on the market you will get to walking barefoot, but they also look like you are wearing monkey feet. To their credit, they have developed a number of new lines with more style over the past ten years, but you will still end up in a conversation about your shoes everywhere you go. Personally, I love mine and wear them for walks, hikes and short runs in the spring and summer. They have been a key ingredient to strengthening my feet, and I recommend them to almost everyone confident enough to wear them in public.

Vivo Barefoot has the best selection of practical, nice-looking barefoot shoes with their Vivo Barefoot line. I use these as work and casual shoes. They have a flat profile and a wide toe box to give your forefoot room. The sole will protect your feet, but you will feel the ground you are walking on. These shoes made me change how I walk. Not having a cushioned heel on them made me realize how much I heel strike and slap my foot as I walk. My heels grew sore and you could hear me walking as my feet slapped the floor. I learned to lean forward slightly to land more on my midfoot; my heels felt better, my feet got stronger, and the slapping stopped.

Merrell teamed up with Vibram to make a super-light hiking and athletic shoe. They have a similar sole to the Five Fingers shoe but are a bit more rugged and don't have the toe slots. If you love the Five Fingers but don't like the monkey-feet look, these are your next best choice. These shoes replaced my Nike Frees as my casual shoe of choice. New Balance and most other brands have followed suit by creating their own minimalist options for running and light hiking, but I encourage people to simply use them as walking shoes and only graduate to running in them if or when their form is ready.

## Plantar fasciitis: An illustrated explanation of why your foot hurts

Plantar fasciitis is a common form of foot pain and one that I find interesting, because it manifests in both active runners as well as relatively sedentary people. How can a person who is training for their third marathon develop the same pain as someone who doesn't exercise much more than walking from their desk to their car? You can't purely blame it on over- or under-use if the desk jockey and the super athlete are experiencing the same problem. What is causing the bottom of people's feet to hurt so much and for so long?

The short answer (a combination of the following factors):

1. The shoes you wear all day (not just while running).

2. Your posture and movement patterns (how you sit, stand, walk, and breathe all day).

3. A nerve irritation in your lower back.

4. Weakness in your feet and tightness in your calves.

5. Fascial restrictions in your visceral system affecting the blood and nerve flow to your feet.

The long answer: It is typically a series of ongoing events that leads to you developing that burning, pulling, aching pain on the bottom of your foot. You may have one or all five of the above issues. If your pain has lasted a long time, it is worth exploring all of them.

## 1. The shoes you wear all day

It is difficult to discuss foot pain without mentioning shoes. All too often, plantar fasciitis gets blamed on a "lack of support," and this bothers me. We are not born wearing shoes, and our feet should not require external pieces of plastic to push our arches up from below. There is a network of muscles, bones and fascia in your feet and calves that have the capacity to support your feet from within. I think it is naive to believe that we can make a foot work better by adding more "support" under the sole. If you track the problem to its origin, I believe that many years of "too much shoe" are to blame more than "not enough support." Once the foot and biomechanics have weakened from too much shoe, more support may feel better in the short term, but you will be doing yourself a disservice in the long term.

My biggest beef with shoes, both causal/dress and running shoes, is the elevated heel. It distorts how the muscles in your feet are supposed to work. It overworks your calves. It encourages overly landing on your heel when you walk and run. It makes it more difficult to control your ankle during heel strike and affects your entire posture, all the way up to your head. Your brain doesn't properly learn how to use your feet, and your body awareness, posture, and movement all suffer.

When your foot and ankle are used to walk on flat ground, the weight of your body is distributed more evenly throughout your entire foot; the muscles in the front of your shin and the bottom of your foot will remain strong at securing the bones in your feet in a firm and supportive position. Conversely, when your foot and ankle are used to having a substantial lift under the heel, your body shifts its center of gravity back and the heel absorbs most of the force. As a result, the muscles in the front of your shin and the bottom of your feet become weak, your forefoot gets floppy and unsupportive and you are a sitting duck to strain your plantar fascia.

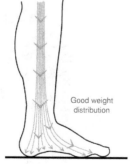

Strong foot that is used to being flat on ground. Forces are distributed evenly throughout the foot.

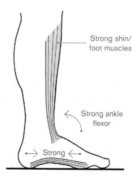

Shin muscles that dorsiflex the ankle stay strong and pair properly with the intrinsic foot muscles to hold the bones of the mid foot together in strong arches.

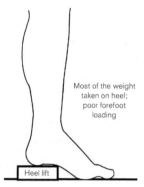

Most of the weight taken on heel; poor forefoot loading

Heel lift

Most of the body's weight taken on the heel. The forefoot hangs down, making it harder for the mid foot bones to lock up in a strong position.

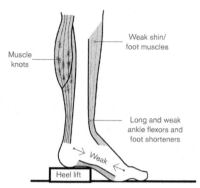

Muscle knots

Weak shin/ foot muscles

Long and weak ankle flexors and foot shorteners

Weak

Heel lift

The shin muscles get long and weak. The intrinsic foot muscles that should help shorten the foot are inhibited, which leads to overactive and overworked calves.

Do you have a floppy foot? Try transitioning to flatter, lighter-profile shoes with a toe box that is wide enough for your forefoot, such as the New Balance Minimus Zero or Merrell Glove.

2. Your posture and movement patterns

Oftentimes, the development of plantar fasciitis takes years and an event becomes the straw that breaks the camel's back to make you start to feel it. Your feet are being squished at the bottom of a tower of moving parts that you must learn to control. How you hold the rest of your body will affect how you load weight onto your feet, and vice-versa. There are many moving parts in your body, but there are only a few centers of control. If you can create some awareness of these four centers, all of the other moving parts will more or less fall into line.

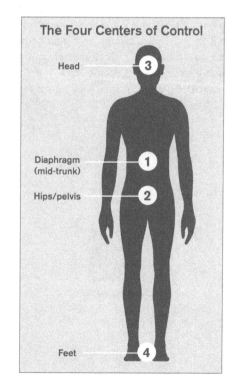

The Four Centers of Control

Head — 3

Diaphragm (mid-trunk) — 1

Hips/pelvis — 2

Feet — 4

For exercise videos related to these four centers, visit WhyThingsHurt.com.

Ideally, your spine has three natural curves, and when you start moving forward your body tilts slightly forward from your ankles and you take a short step. If you have good posture and move well, your center of gravity will be largely over-top of your foot as it hits the ground, and your ankle will be in a good position to help push you forward.

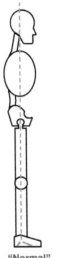
**"Normal"**
Weight balanced down through the body

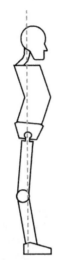
**Back gripper**
Uneven weight distribution

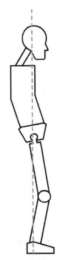
**Stomach gripper**
Uneven weight distribution

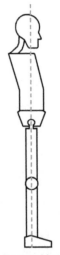
**Butt and back gripper/compressor**
Weight shifted to back line of body

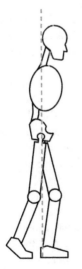
**Normal walking**
Slight forward lean from ankle and weight over foot at impact

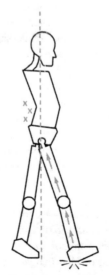
**Back gripper walking**
Increased heel impact and weight behind foot at impact, creating a jarring force with every step

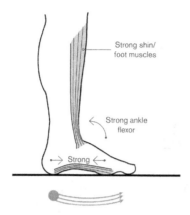

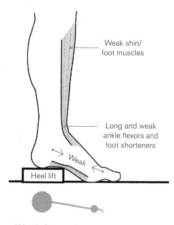

**Strong foot + good posture =**
the forces through the foot become like a
rocker to transfer you forward

**Weak foot + bad posture =**
big impact force on heel, the forefoot slaps down
with little control, and little propulsion is created

Many people, unfortunately, become too "back grippy," in their attempt to "stand up straight" and actually end up tipping their torso backward. A back-gripping posture tends to shift your center of gravity back toward your heels and will make you prone to having a floppy forefoot (see picture above). I liken trying to walk or run forward while your torso is tipped backward to driving with your E-brake on: things will wear down, and you are working harder than you have to. When your upper body is leaning backward as you walk, your leg will tend to stride further out in front of you and your heel will impact the ground ahead of your body instead of underneath it; this will effectively create a harmful impact instead of a weight transfer and make you pull yourself along instead of pushing yourself forward. The cumulative effect of walking or running with poor mechanics will beat up your heel and your plantar fascia.

Good posture and mechanics requires the foot to act as a rocker for weight transfer to help propel you forward when walking or running. For a person with poor posture and weak feet, the foot endures a forceful impact on the heel, then the forefoot slaps down and little propulsion is created. Your feet are tough structures, but over time this repetitive trauma builds up and your body becomes aggravated. If you want to feel what it's like to get support and propulsion from your feet, watch the "toe spreader" tape job video on WhyThingsHurt.com.

Even though your mid back is a long way from your foot pain, addressing the posture and mobility of your torso can go a long way to improving your stride, and it will take much of the force off your feet. I will touch on this further in the next section, and there are numerous videos on WhyThingsHurt.com to demonstrate the concepts.

## 3. A nerve irritation in your lower back

Your nerves are the electrical wiring of your body, and your L5 and S1 nerve roots from the small of your back supply the electrical wiring to your feet; if you irritate these nerves, you are just as likely to experience foot pain as you are to experience back pain. Foot pain can come almost exclusively from your back, even if your back itself doesn't bother you; it is called "referred pain," and it is a common ingredient to persistent plantar fasciitis.

The faulty postures, movement mechanics, and impact forces discussed above can all create compressive forces on your lower back. If your upper body is leaning backward, it is more than likely to create a compressive extension hinge in your lower back as you stand, walk and run. Over time, the compression in your lower back will irritate the L5/S1 nerve roots, which are major feeders to your sciatic nerve which extends right down to your heel. When nerves are irritated, they will create bands of tension and knots in the muscles that they innervate—in this case, your foot and calf. When muscles are full of bands of tension, they become stiff and act functionally weak. Stiffness in the calf and lack of muscular support in the foot leaves the plantar fascia vulnerable to strain and injury; it will lower the threshold of what it takes to create pain.

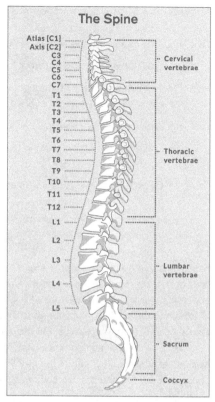

**The Spine**

Atlas [C1]
Axis [C2]
C3
C4
C5
C6
C7
— Cervical vertebrae

T1
T2
T3
T4
T5
T6
T7
T8
T9
T10
T11
T12
— Thoracic vertebrae

L1
L2
L3
L4
L5
— Lumbar vertebrae

— Sacrum

— Coccyx

Compression and degeneration of spinal vertebrae can cause nerve irritations which affect the structures, organs, and functions elsewhere in the body, such as your feet.

If nerve root irritation is a major part of your plantar fasciitis (as it usually is), it typically responds quite well to treatment with intramuscular stimulation (IMS). Treating the hips, lower spine, calves, and the muscle in the bottom of your feet, although uncomfortable, can create almost immediate relief. The challenge then becomes to correct your posture and movement mechanics so you stop irritating your lower back—otherwise the problem will slowly arise again. There is a good sequence of exercises to follow on WhyThingsHurt.com to help correct your posture and movement. If your feet are quite painful, the toe spreader tape job mentioned above is a great way to offload your foot and give your strained plantar fascia a rest.

4. Weakness in your feet and tightness in your calves

I will keep this one short and summarize what you have already read:

- Traditional shoes do the work for your feet and inevitably create weakness.
- The compensations that occur due to poor posture, shoes, and weak feet cause the calves to get overworked and tight.
- Irritation in the nerves in your back causes your calves to tighten further.
- There is a direct relationship between calf tightness and forefoot weakness/floppiness.
- Calve tightness + foot weakness = eventual foot pain.

5. Fascial restriction in your visceral system affecting the nerve and blood flow to your feet

Fascia is a thin connective tissue found throughout your body that helps support and hold everything together. Your visceral system is referring to all of your organs in your abdominal cavity and trunk. Organs like your intestines, stomach, liver, and kidneys all attach to the back wall of your abdominal cavity. They are loosely held in place by fascia, ligaments, and pressure, but they need to be able to freely slide over each other to allow normal human movement. Issues like stress, trauma, pregnancy and abdominal surgeries can affect the mobility of specific areas of your visceral system. These mobility restrictions can cause alignment issues and irritate or impede blood and nerve flow.

The major nerves and blood vessels to your lower body pass through your pelvis en route to your feet, and as such, fascial restrictions in the lower abdomen can be responsible for foot and ankle pain. Personally, I have found that having visceral manipulation on either end of my large intestine (cecum and sigmoid colon) to have a significant impact on the blood flow and mobility in my feet. Clinically, I have found that almost all of my clients who have improved but plateaued with IMS and postural work have found the missing link to their foot or leg issues to be visceral in origin.

It seems difficult to believe that your guts not moving well is the reason why your feet have hurt for three months, but when you understand the anatomy of it, it makes sense. Resistant plantar fasciitis is usually multifaceted in origin, but your organs can certainly be one of the culprits.

# Tennis Players: World Champions to Social Butterflies

Tennis has to be the most social sport that I have been exposed to over the years, and one of the few that I never truly embraced, even though I had ample opportunity as a kid. My father was the tennis and badminton coach for the top boys' private school in Vancouver, and my mother was a national-level badminton player, so racket sports were seemingly in my genes. I grew up watching Boris Becker, Andre Agassi, and Pete Sampras with my dad, but I always gravitated to team sports for myself.

As a physiotherapist who had just learned everything there was to know about golf, I was looking to broaden my horizons, and tennis was a natural shift because, as I learned, many of the professionals and retirees that I was treating also played tennis. I ended up taking a top-down approach for building my caseload with tennis players by connecting with the local pro at Vancouver's biggest tennis club. He was one of the top Masters-level players in the city, and with his endorsement came a cohort of working professionals in their forties, fifties, and sixties who also represented Canada in the World Championships every year. It was great to be exposed to a group of people who had been lifelong athletes and who were still playing at an elite level, despite having busy lives. It was inspiring to see that there were parents who returned to their sports after surviving the pressures of work and parenting, as I was going down the rabbit hole of three kids in three years.

After a few years, tennis players began to dominate my caseload much more than golfers, because I took the advice of then-CEO of Tennis BC: "Connect with the women and don't waste your time with the men. If you get the women, they will send the men." It was true, and it worked. I started to appreciate just how much socializing surrounded tennis, and that women talked to each other a lot, and about everything. I became the physiotherapist for three cohorts of tennis players in Vancouver: the aging elite, the working professionals and the wealthy wives who seemed to know everybody and seemingly lived at their clubs. It was the right mix of people to know and a great group of people to work with that became the word-of-mouth engine that allowed my business to thrive.

Tennis is a sport that people can—and do—play throughout life. I have worked with elite teenagers all the way up to a man who competed in the over-seventy-five category at the World Championships, and every age group seems to be prone to over-training. If there has been one group that I have had to stress the concept of "less is more" to, it has been tennis players, particularly the aging ones, because their bodies can only take so much before they start to break down.

The top five problems that tend to bring tennis players into physiotherapy for servicing are:

1. Tennis elbow

2. Shoulder pain and rotator cuff impingements

3. Knee pain

4. Lower back pain

5. Torn calf/Achilles

## 1. Tennis elbow

Tennis elbow and golfer's elbow are the typical names given to elbow pain; tennis being pain on the outside of the elbow, and golf being pain on the inside of the elbow. The more technical term is lateral epicondylitis, which simply indicates tendonitis in a specific location. Putting a name to elbow pain doesn't help you to get rid of it, but understanding why it happens and where it comes from will.

Tendons are the tough bits of tissue that attach muscle to bones, and tendonitis literally means inflammation of the tendon. This term can be misleading when it comes to elbow pain, because many people have pain that persists for months in the complete absence of swelling and inflammation. That is because elbow pain is not only an overuse injury. It happens when the muscles in use are in an irritable state due to a nerve irritation stemming from your neck and shoulder. Nerves are the electrical wiring of muscles, and when they are irritated, it doesn't take much to overuse the muscles and tendons that they innervate, resulting in inflammation and pain. If you rest the joint, the body will heal the inflammation, but the nerve irritation may persist and thus the inflammation and pain will return as soon as you attempt to use your arm again.

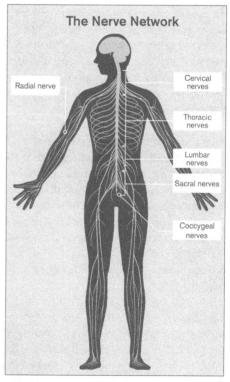

The radial nerve extends from the base of the neck, through the shoulder, and down to the elbow.

Muscles are comprised of stringy tissue that can stretch and contract. The muscle should have a certain amount of resting tone in it; for example, at rest it is slightly contracted, not flaccid or extremely tense, which is dictated by the input of the nerve. If the nerve is irritated as it extends from the spine, or anywhere in the periphery, it will result in an altered signal reaching the muscle. This altered signal can create bands of tension in the muscle, which will strain the joint and the tendons and will likely create pain. Muscles are attached to bones on either side of a joint by tendons. Tendons are a tougher tissue in that they only stretch a small amount; when the muscle is in a banded state, the tendons endure much more stress and strain when the joint is used, and the result is typically tendonitis.

Here is a simple illustration to demonstrate a joint in a healthy, normal state. The muscle is resting in a gently contracted state with some elasticity between the two tendon attachments to the bones on either end. The nerve is supplying a steady signal from the spinal cord, and the joint should move freely and be pain free.

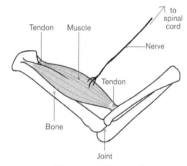

**Normal state muscle**

Conversely, below we see an illustration of a joint in a painful state due to and underlying nerve irritation. Something has annoyed the nerve, which is causing it to send an altered signal to the muscle. Imagine a flickering light bulb in a lamp when the wiring is off. The annoyed nerve causes the muscle to create bands of tension like muscle knots. The knots are typically tender to the touch and the area can be colder due to poor blood flow through the tightened muscles. The increased tension in the muscle will compress the joint, ultimately leading to pain and potential degeneration over time. It can even make the bones feel bruised from the constant tug of the tendons.

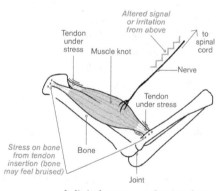

**Irritated nerve causing tension**

Postural issues that create immobility in the upper back tend to lead to an extension hinge in the lower part of the neck. This causes the person to move far too much through the C5, 6 and 7 joints, which can irritate the nerve roots as they extend from the spine. It doesn't always create neck pain but can simply annoy the nerve and lower the threshold for what it takes to overuse it further down the chain.

The C6 and 7 nerve roots are the electrical wiring for your lats, biceps, and triceps, as well as the muscles in your forearm; if the neck is irritated, these muscles will hold tension. Postural imbalances and movement mechanics related to certain sports and occupations can also lead to tightness in these muscle groups. It is this combination of neck irritation and repeated movement patterns that can make elbow pain last indefinitely. That is why neck and muscle irritation must be dealt with first, followed by postural correction. If you only treat the elbow pain, you are addressing the symptoms and not the root cause.

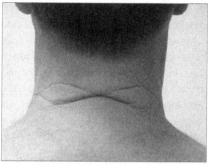

Postural issues that create immobility in the upper back tend to lead to an extension hinge in the lower part of the neck; this can appear as a crease in the neck, as shown.

Many people will attempt to stretch and strengthen the forearm muscles with limited success, because the root cause of the problem is not in the forearm. In fact, overly stretching and exercising the elbow while it is in an irritable state may make it worse. The best course of treatment for sub-acute to chronic elbow pain is to first use IMS (intramuscular stimulation) on the neck, shoulder, and arm, then progress to postural and movement awareness of the upper back, neck, and shoulder.

IMS can significantly calm down the nerve irritation and pain to open a window for you to address your posture and movement problems that created the issue in the first place. The results of IMS can last for quite a long time, but if you continue your faulty habits, you are likely to re-irritate the nerves, muscles, and tendons. Icing and resting the elbow alone won't suffice, because it only addresses the symptoms. Attempting to stretch and strengthen the forearm muscles tends to be a waste of time. IMS alone will work better, but again, it won't be a permanent solution, because you can re-aggravate it. The best option is a combination of rest and ice initially, followed by IMS, and finally, posture and movement awareness exercises.

## 2. Shoulder pain and rotator cuff impingements

Your shoulder is brilliantly designed to allow your arm to reach, grab, throw, push, and pull, but if you have experienced shoulder pain you might argue that there are some flaws in the blueprints. I have seen shoulder pain bring some of the toughest guys to their knees and frozen shoulders put women's lives on hold for one to two years. I, personally, have dislocated my shoulder multiple times and eventually had surgery on it in 2001. My shoulders and I are not friends, but I have learned how to keep my enemies close and under control.

Knowing what I know about biomechanics and anatomy, I still support the idea that the shoulder is extraordinarily designed, but it should come with a detailed instruction manual of how to use it properly. Your shoulder is a complex ball-in-socket joint, with its function intimately tied to the posture and alignment of your rib cage and thoracic spine. "Normal" movement in your shoulder requires the ball to spin in the socket, the shoulder blade to slide over your rib cage, and your torso to remain in a relatively stable position; a problem in any or all of these factors will lead to dysfunction and eventually pain in your shoulder.

It is simple to determine what structure in your shoulder may be damaged and hurting, but it can be more difficult to understand why you damaged anything in the first place. That said, sometimes the "why" is easy: you may have tried tackling a two-hundred-pound Kiwi rugby player determined to run through you and your shoulder lost the battle (like mine did), but most of the time "why" is more complex than you would like. Shoulder pain usually involves a combination of factors that, over time, lead to the insidious onset of pain.

Top five factors related to persistent shoulder pain (the "why"):

1. Poor posture in the mid-upper back:
   - Too hunched forward.
   - Too braced backward.
2. Poor muscle balance around the shoulder girdle (tightness and weakness).
3. Poor awareness of proper shoulder blade-trunk stability.
4. Poor movement patterns developed from sport or during childhood.
5. Alignment and stability issues in your upper ribs.

Top five painful/irritated/damaged structures due to the above factors (the "what"):

1. Rotator cuff impingements.
2. Biceps tendonitis.
3. Strain in the muscles from the shoulder to the neck.
4. Tension on the nerves from the neck to the shoulder.
5. Bursitis.

How the above "whys" combine to create the above "whats":

When you lift your arm over your head, it may reach 180 degrees; about 120 degrees of this movement should happen in the ball-and-socket part of your shoulder, and about 60 degrees is accomplished by your shoulder blade sliding upward on your rib cage. Most shoulder problems arise when something restricts the proper movement of your shoulder blade. Having a rounded upper back will naturally tip your shoulder blades too far forward. Having a flat upper back may allow your shoulder blades to rest too low on your trunk. Having a swayback and overactivity of your lats will cause your shoulders to sit too low and restrict the upward movement of your shoulder blade.

When you attempt to lift your arm and the shoulder blade is either starting in a bad place or not moving well, you will force too much movement upon the ball-in-socket joint and are more likely to pinch or rub sensitive muscles or tendons. Your rotator cuff isn't one structure, but four muscles that work together to help hold the ball in the socket; these muscles (as well as your bicep) turn into tendons and attach all around your shoulder. Pinching these tendons under one of the bones of your shoulder blade, called your acromion, is the most common cause of acute shoulder pain and is referred to as a rotator cuff impingement.

Acutely pinching a tendon in your shoulder can be very painful and can result from one specific incident, or over time by moving poorly and repeatedly rubbing a tendon, creating too much friction. The latter can lead to tendonitis or bursitis in your shoulder; "-itis" is simply a suffix meaning "inflammation of"—tendonitis is inflammation of the tendon and bursitis is inflammation of the bursa. The bursa is a thin fluid-filled sac around most major joints, much like the air bags for your joints. If you start developing too much friction by moving poorly, they swell up and become inflamed; resting and icing them helps, but you have to fix the movement problem for permanent relief.

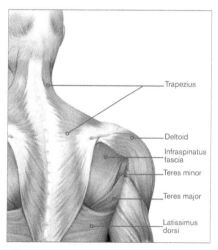

Trapezius

Deltoid

Infraspinatus fascia

Teres minor

Teres major

Latissimus dorsi

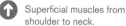

Superficial muscles from shoulder to neck.

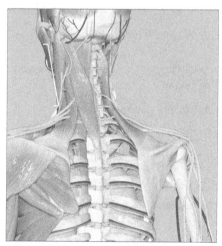

Nerves and deep muscles from neck to shoulder.

The neck is closely linked to the shoulder by muscles and nerves. There are a number of muscles that attach your shoulder up to your neck, and it is common for persistent shoulder problems to irritate the neck and compound the problem. The nerves that extend from your mid to lower neck are the electrical wiring for all the muscles in your shoulder and arm, so if they become annoyed you will likely feel referred pain and muscle tension in your shoulder, arm, and even your fingers. Nervy arm pain will only further degrade your movement patterns and can start a vicious cycle of your shoulder irritating your neck and your neck irritating your arm; if this is the case, calming down the neck irritation should become priority one.

Following the process of release, re-educate, rebuild is the best way to fix most shoulder problems with lasting results. If you have reached the point of feeling pain, you likely have a handful of muscles that have tightened up and are making "normal" movement challenging or even impossible; releasing these muscles is an important first step to decreasing pain and restoring movement. I have found that IMS is the best way to release the bracing muscles around a joint. Once muscles have been released, pain is often significantly improved and movement becomes easier. Establishing proper movement and control of your shoulder is what I mean by re-educate, and it is the key to preventing shoulder problems from surfacing again. If you spend the time addressing your posture and arm movements before attempting further strengthening, you will get to where you want to be faster and will end up functionally stronger. Once the movement dysfunctions are corrected, shoulder, core, and general body strengthening exercises can be helpful for prevention and performance of your arm.

### 3. Knee pain

I have heard countless tennis players complain that knees were just poorly designed. In fact, they are designed quite well, but they are at the mercy of your hips and your ankles. Your knee is a big hinge joint built to flex and extend, while your hips and ankles are built to twist and roll. When your feet become weak and your hips tighten up, your knees are left in a vulnerable position. Tennis requires a fair amount of court mobility with planting, pushing off, and changing directions. Acutely, these plant-and-twist movements can result in a tear of the meniscus, or more chronically can lead to patellofemoral syndrome, bursitis, or even osteoarthritis. No matter what structure is hurting, physiotherapy can help by freeing up the deep muscles in your hips and thighs, checking your alignment and helping you strengthen your feet. You would be amazed how much better you can move around the court after having IMS performed on your hips and legs, even with an arthritic knee.

### 4. Lower-back pain

Lower-back pain in tennis players is typically due to compression and torsion. Your lower back is built to flex and extend, and, just like your knees, it hates twisting, rotational forces upon it. Your lumbar spine is sandwiched between your hips, which are built to rotate, and your thoracic spine, which is also built to rotate. The flexibility and control of your trunk and your hips will dictate how much or how little back pain you experience. Court agility and power should come from how well you load your hips and how well you stabilize your trunk. If you are either too stiff or too mobile in either area, your back will experience problems. Seeing a physiotherapist to release the tight structures that are causing the pain, to teach you how to move properly in your hips and trunk, and to then work on creating strength in your new movements is the best way to create long-term health for your back as a tennis player.

## 5. Torn calf/Achilles tendons

Back-pedaling on the court is the best way to strain your calves. A quick step back and change in direction puts a large amount of force on your calves and Achilles, which under normal circumstances they should be able to sustain. However, if your lower back and hips are quite tight, you likely have a moderate amount of annoyance happening to your sciatic nerve (it is the electrical wiring to most of the muscles down the back of your leg). Ongoing irritation of your sciatic nerve will create subtle muscle knots and bands of tension in your hamstrings and calves that make the muscles less flexible and less tolerant of sudden stretching forces. The combination of back and hip tension in an active, aging tennis player makes calf strains very common occurrences, particularly in men. It is the same mechanism of injury for a moderate muscle tear and a full-blown Achilles tendon rupture. The calf strain may lay you up for two to six weeks while the Achilles rupture can keep you out for a year. It should be good motivation to keep your hips loose. Again, the best way to treat these strains is IMS in the back, hips, and calves. Once the pain has calmed down, it is important to learn how to squat, move laterally, and push off again—properly, this time.

# Take Aways and Resources

**Take Aways**

→ Sports become part of who you are from a young age. Embrace your past as you try to control your future.

→ Working on your "core" is more than abdominal strength. It is about developing controlled and coordinated movement for light or heavy tasks, for power or finesse.

→ Exercising has physical and mental implications. Ask yourself why you are doing what you do and set goals for yourself.

→ Lack of flexibility is not directly proportional to a lack of stretching. Move well, stretch less.

→ We are not born wearing shoes, and our feet are not designed to be externally supported by orthotics and cushy shoes. Learn to use your feet.

**Websites:**

✦ FitGolf.com: the company that started me down the path of working with golfers.

✦ VivoBarefoot.com: my favorite minimalist shoes that I wear to work every day.

# Respecting and Correcting Your Mother

## Myths to Dispel:

- "Stand up straight, shoulders back and down" is good advice

- Just because you can stand, sit, walk, and breathe means you are good at it

- A woman's body will naturally recover after pregnancy

# Everything Your Mother Taught You About Posture is Wrong

Most people think of posture simply as the need to keep your chest up and your shoulders back and down. Sounds like a simple feat, right? Then why will most people admit that they believe they have bad posture? The answer is because good posture is not a simple thing, it is actually a learned, coordinated skill that encompasses the entire body. We are what we repeatedly do, and our posture is a reflection of our childhood, our sports, our jobs, our emotions, and our attitudes.

There is a continuum of flexibility and mobility among the population. Some people are naturally loose-jointed and hypermobile, while others are compressed and stiff as a board. Where you end up on the spectrum seems to be partly genetic and partly due to personality. The people who fall in the middle tend to have the least pain and fewest injuries. The further a person strays in either direction from the average, the more posture, movement, and pain problems they tend to develop. There is not one perfect posture for everybody, but there is a norm that we should all try to achieve, no matter which side of normal we are on.

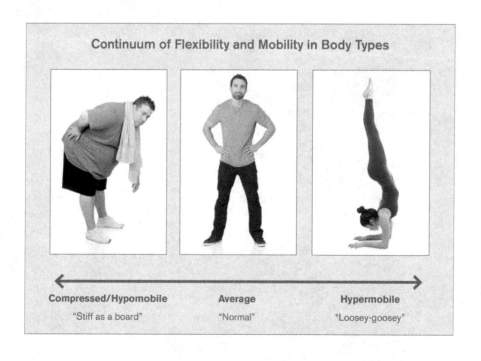

**Continuum of Flexibility and Mobility in Body Types**

| Compressed/Hypomobile | Average | Hypermobile |
|---|---|---|
| "Stiff as a board" | "Normal" | "Loosey-goosey" |

Our bodies are brilliantly built to deal with gravity as a constant downward force, but most people don't know how to use their bodies properly or efficiently, and end up with muscle imbalances, pain, and dysfunction in attempt to stay upright. Posture should be considered a life skill and not a genetic trait that we can blame on our parents. A basic understanding of anatomy and biomechanics can save people a great deal of grief throughout life.

Here you can see a model of a spine, pelvis, and hips. The skeleton is the structural foundation of your body, and it is built for both stability and mobility. Weight is distributed down your spinal column, to your sacrum, through your sacroiliac (SI) joints, into your hips, down to your knees and out your ankles and feet. All of these joints allow us to move freely, but if we want to carry something or push something heavy, we need to use our muscles to properly line up our skeleton in order to distribute load and create stability. This is the concept that most people fail to understand, and is the basis of having good posture for standing, sitting, walking, and higher-level activities.

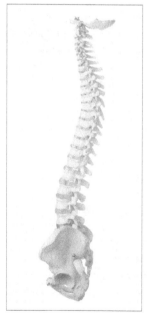
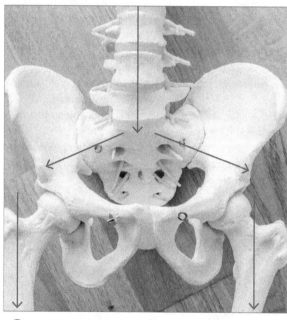

 Model of pelvis and spine.　　 Model of spine, SI joints, pelvis, and hips.

For what we consider "normal" posture and good stability, the pelvis should be slightly tipped forward; there should be a slight inward curve in your lower back; a gently rounded curve from the top of your lower back to your neck; and another inward curve in your neck. Your ears should be over your shoulders, and your arms should hang relaxed down the midline of your torso.

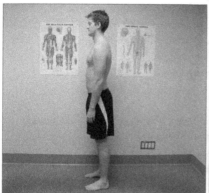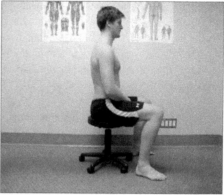

⬆ Good standing and sitting posture. Standing and sitting properly are skills that should be learned.

Our bodies are inherently lazy and will usually take the path of least resistance when it comes to moving and dealing with gravity. Over time, we usually develop specific muscle imbalances that pull us in one direction or another away from the ideal "normal" posture. This process begins when we are young children, and becomes strongly ingrained by the influence and effects of our parents, friends, sports, emotions, shoes, and injuries. Some muscles tend to become quite strong and tight, while others become long and weak, which can make it more challenging to effectively stack and balance your skeleton. The result is that we tend to hang off of certain joints and ligaments instead of using postural muscles to hold us up. It is this practice that results in most chronic pain issues; your body starts being controlled by gravity instead of you, and you end up stretching ligaments, compressing joints, overworking muscles, and generally feeling sore and tight all the time.

The area where most people tend to go wrong with their posture is how they attempt to balance their upper body on their lower body. The pelvis should be balanced on the hips by two large ball-and-socket joints. These joints have available movement in all directions, so if you have overly flexible hips, it can be challenging to effectively balance your upper body on your lower body. You often see this with young girls and people who have done a lot of yoga, dance, and gymnastics. Ask them to stand in one place for a while, and you will see them jut out a hip to one side, cross their legs or hang their pelvis forward, because they can't figure out how to vertically stack their spine. The usual strategy is then to use their back, spine, and shoulders by lifting their chest, pulling their shoulders back and down, and hyperextending their knees. This group will end up with chronically tight back and shoulders and will have vulnerable knees because they are only using their back, thighs, and spine. Figuring out how to use their hamstrings, butt, and abs together would do them a world of good.

On the other hand, some people go too far in the other direction. They develop tight hips and make up for the lack of hip movement with too much back movement. Forces and loads that should be transferred through the big, tough hip joints end up beating

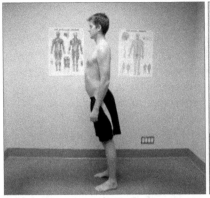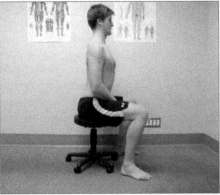

⬆ Those who stand braced tend to sit braced as well.

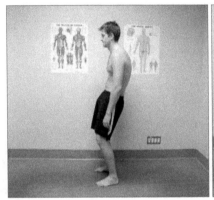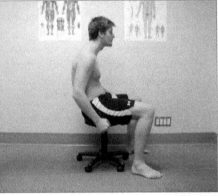

⬆ Those who stand with their butt tucked forward often sit this way.

up on the joints and ligaments of the lower back and knees. The relative tension required to move in the stiff hips is much more than it takes to move through the loose spine, so the person subconsciously takes the plane of least resistance and the spine takes the beating. This is a common phenomenon throughout the body, and it is what I call the "tail that wags the dog" syndrome. Peripheral joints stiffen up, making it easier to move in the spine instead.

This is the concept that core stability tries to correct: learning to keep your spine in a good position while you move. Unfortunately, people often think this is necessary only for growing stronger, but in reality it is a skill that you first need to learn before you can work toward strengthening. Attempts at strengthening your core before you understand how to use it properly usually ends up strengthening only your muscle imbalances, which is why people often get hurt at the gym.

Your upper back is the stiffest part of your spine and the part that tends to round the most on some people. It is supposed to be slightly rounded, but when it starts going too far, it will push your head forward. Our brains have a head-righting reflex that tries to keep our eyes looking straight forward, and our mothers have a tendency to tell us "chest up, shoulders back and down." The combination of these factors often causes most people to lean backward when attempting to stand up straight. The mid and lower back have less relative tension than the upper back, so most attempts to stand up straight end up tipping your upper torso backward instead of straightening out the curved upper back. This, in turn, usually causes the pelvis to push forward and the head to move relatively forward. It looks good from the front, but if you turn to look at your side profile, you may be in for a surprise. It is this postural concept that creates a lot of pain and stiffness. It is also related to the hump you can develop at the base of your neck, the bulge in your lower stomach you can't get rid of, and the bunions on your feet you thought were genetic.

Torso posture and shoulder posture are two separate entities; addressing the torso is more important than addressing the shoulders when trying to create lasting change.

WhyThingsHurt.com has a good video titled "Everything Your Mother Taught You About Posture is Wrong" to help you understand these concepts and to help you gain an appreciation for how challenging and uncommon good posture actually is.

# My Mother: The Art of Fixing Mom

My mother is a loving, compassionate person with some very intriguing personality traits that I'm sure are partly responsible for molding who I am. She has these polarized characteristics that will make you shake your head and be impressed at the same time. She was an elite-level badminton player and PE teacher—two activities that require agility and athleticism—but she is quite clumsy and generally has poor body awareness. She excelled in leadership and became the CEO of both Sport BC and KidSport Canada, but in her heart she held many insecurities. She is well read, well-traveled, and politically engaged, but she is a lighthearted goof who mispronounces simple words and doesn't take herself too seriously. She has strong beliefs and is willing to work harder than most to achieve what she believes in, but fixing her ailing body after sixty years of physical trauma and cognitive neglect has been one of her most complex challenges to work through, not to mention mine.

Treating friends and family as a physiotherapist comes with a unique challenge, because they don't see me as "Brent the professional"; they see me as the child they raised, or the guy they hang out with on Saturday nights. They trust me to help fix them, but they are less inclined to listen to my advice about changing their own behavior because of our relationship. The experiences of treating my parents, my friends, and my wife have shown me how much of a cognitive role is present in a therapeutic relationship, which does not work very well when it is complicated by a deep personal relationship. I've learned that I can do things to my family, but I am best to have others teach them what they should do for themselves. I become an impatient teacher, and they become inattentive or overly sensitive students because of our history together. I'm sure this phenomenon is not exclusive to me, because we all want to help our families, but they are the quickest ones to get under our skin.

If there was a gene for being injury prone, my mom got it and passed it on to me. I remember being a little kid at the waterslides and seeing my mom waiting to climb the ladder out of the pool, only to have the child in front of her jump off backward and almost break her nose, filling the pool with blood. I've heard stories about her trying to demonstrate something to her PE class on the gymnastics rings and actually getting stuck in them, hanging from the ceiling until another teacher came and saved her. She also pounded the hell out of her feet playing competitive badminton for half of her life until she saw a couple of orthopedic surgeons who claimed to be able to fix them, but three surgeries later she only developed new pains and new problems in her feet.

One of the nuances of being a physiotherapist is that when anyone hurts themselves or has pain in your social circle, somehow it becomes your problem too. Some people genuinely want help and advice while others just tell me about their pain as a form of small talk because they know what I do for a living. My mom has resided in both groups over the years and has come to me for help on and off while trying to not interfere with my daily business. She has struggled with her feet, her hips, her back, neck and shoulder, but would only make a point of coming to see me on occasions when it became really bad. I was always happy to help, but I started to realize we weren't getting anywhere because our visits were too few and far between. We were treating her pain and not her real problems: her posture and movement patterns.

My mom is a long-standing back gripper with poor awareness of her feet, competitive tendencies, and impulsive movement patterns. Her back muscles are thick, strong, and tight, and her deep hip muscles are so overworked and tender that she yelps if you even lightly touch the prominent bone on the side of her hip. Using intramuscular stimulation (IMS) on her hips, back, lats, and traps always gave her relief, but she would inevitably be back with the same problem a month or two later, so I decided to tackle her posture and movement patterns.

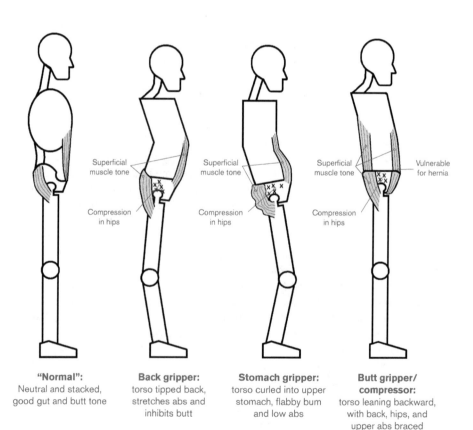

"Normal":
Neutral and stacked, good gut and butt tone

Back gripper:
torso tipped back, stretches abs and inhibits butt

Stomach gripper:
torso curled into upper stomach, flabby bum and low abs

Butt gripper/ compressor:
torso leaning backward, with back, hips, and upper abs braced

I tried to teach her how to open up the lower-back part of her rib cage, to breathe differently, and walk differently. I tried to help her to develop body awareness, but I found out a few years later from my sister that she stopped coming to see me because she felt that I was being mean to her. She still came occasionally for IMS, but she had also found a Pilates instructor who resonated with her. She tried some classes, but the instructor called out her competitiveness and suggested she instead try one-on-one sessions. She stuck with this instructor for a number of years and continued to give me excited updates on all this fascinating body awareness she was developing. I was thrilled with her happiness and that we had found someone who she would comfortably listen to. She was making her body a priority for the first time in her life and was blown away by what she could and couldn't do. It was the right place for her to connect her physical and cognitive worlds that had been living separate lives for a long time.

After a few years of Pilates, as well as intermittent IMS and visceral manipulation from me, my mom was still experiencing life-impacting foot pain. She looked into seeing doctors again, tried orthotics and new shoes, but she never officially asked for my advice. It was always the occasional visit here or there with no continuity. I finally confronted her, and she told me that she knew that I was busy and didn't want to cost me money by taking a time slot in my day. I explained to her that making sure that my mother could walk was more important to me than a bit of money each week and encouraged her to start seeing me with some regularity instead of talking to another surgeon about her feet.

We decided that she needed something more functional than Pilates to help her stop pounding her feet until she couldn't walk. Pilates prepared her to connect to her body and to be open to moving differently, but it wasn't translating into a change in her gait, so I referred her to an experienced kinesiologist in my office for gait training and functional movement patterns, all in the vertical position. She committed to improving her body and visited me once a week for IMS on her hips, back, and calves, and visceral manipulation on her heart and lungs. She switched her shoes and tried orthotics again, and then diligently worked with the kinesiologist until her foot pain was under control. She still has bad feet and less-than-ideal posture, but her commitment to attend to her body has empowered her to manage her problems and has substantially decreased her pain. I stuck to my role of working on her and pointed her in the direction of others who could guide her more effectively than I could, and from that point forward her strong work ethic made the difference.

My mom is a good example of how behavior affects pain, and the importance of making a commitment to your own needs. I have seen countless grandmothers and grandfathers who have written off their bodies because their doctor showed them an X-ray displaying some degeneration, but I have also surprised just as many by helping them reach a point of no pain, even though their joints aren't in great shape. People forget what "normal" is supposed to feel like after their bodies have been stiff and in pain for a long time, but I have found that decompressing them with IMS can provide a glimpse into normalcy and the motivation to attend to their bodies in a new way.

Maintenance and prevention are even more important when you get older, but most people believe that they are too old to change and just live with their pain. I have seen people eliminate decade-old pains and substantially improve how they move; it just took a commitment to themselves.

# Pregnancy, Pain, and Posture: Restoring Normal Movement

I will concede right off the bat that I am not a woman and have never been pregnant. That said, I have worked with and treated women at all stages of pregnancy, including immediately after C-sections and women who, twenty years later, are still trying to get their bodies back. From what I have seen, there is no other experience a person can go through that is more physically and mentally challenging on your body than getting pregnant, having the baby, and making it through the first five years in one piece.

Medicine has come a long way in ensuring mother and baby are physiologically healthy from conception through to the birth, but there still remains a significant lack of proper support and education for women when it comes to pain, posture, movement, and physical function both during and after pregnancy. The most important factor to consider is that most women don't have great posture, movement mechanics, or strength before they get pregnant, so this issue is not solely created by pregnancy but merely exposed by it. Most women are not used to carrying around ten to thirty pounds all day, having to bend and pick up things from the floor sixty times a day or hunching over while breast feeding time and time again. These are physical demands that would be hard on anyone, but particularly trying on someone whose body has changed so dramatically in a relatively short period of time and is functioning on very little sleep.

Ideally, to move well in order to prevent pain and dysfunction, you need to be able to vertically stack your body in good posture as you stand, sit, push, pull, walk, and lift. The strength and stability in your muscles and joints, combined with your body awareness, are the main factors to help you maintain good posture throughout the day. As your pregnancy progresses, your abdominals continue to stretch and get proportionately weaker. At the same time, you are growing heavier and your joints are getting looser due to hormonal factors. The strategy your body used to use in order to keep you vertical will fundamentally start to change, because you now have a weak, heavy belly pulling you forward; other muscle groups must pick up the slack.

As a woman's center of gravity shifts forward during pregnancy, her back and glute muscles should ideally work harder in order to keep her vertical and walking relatively normally, but her body will be fantastic at cheating and does whatever feels easiest to move at the time. The result is usually to lean most of the torso backward and to place both hands on the lower back and hips for support. The trouble is that when you stand or walk around with your pelvis in front of your feet, instead of over-top of them, your glutes cannot function properly, and the deep muscles in your hips and groin become tight, overworked and sore. This poor posture is the primary cause for women getting SI (sacroiliac) joint pain, pubic bone pain, and sciatica during and after pregnancy.

The best thing a woman can do to prepare herself physically for pregnancy is to create body awareness of how to stand, sit, walk, and lift mechanically well before her body starts to change. It is much easier to find your way back after pregnancy if you know where you started from—most women don't. Most new moms turn into a "butt gripper" or "back gripper." Their bodies have been so stretched out that they will subconsciously grip and clench certain muscle groups to hold everything together, while trying to perform the physical job of being a mom. The trouble is that the muscles they are gripping and clenching are supposed to be moving muscles, and when you ask a big, moving muscle to be both a passive stabilizer and a mover at the same time, something inevitably breaks down. This is where body awareness becomes the most important factor as it relates to life tasks like standing, breathing, and bending.

You cannot move well if you tend to brace major muscle groups during light-load activities, and you cannot be functionally strong if you cannot move well. The best preventative tool and the first rehabilitative step should be to learn how to turn off some muscles before you attempt to turn on a bunch of new ones. The post-pregnancy education for women tends to overly focus on practicing pelvic-floor exercises like kegels. These exercises are useful to help restore and activate important muscles, but they are only a small piece of the puzzle when it comes to restoring a woman's posture, movement, and physique. A woman can diligently do kegels every day, all day, and still end up with pelvic pain, weakness, and incontinence if she doesn't learn to stop squeezing and bracing muscles in her trunk and bum when she stands up.

The trunk and pelvis create a cavity inside for all your organs to function and move. This cavity is a system under pressure, and if you squeeze it, the contents will look for the easiest place to escape. In pregnant women and new moms, the two places the contents are going to push are the center line of the stomach muscles called the linea alba and the pelvic floor. If enough pressure is exerted on the linea alba, it can tear and create a diastasis, which is effectively an abdominal hernia splitting your six-pack muscle down the middle. If enough pressure is pushed downward on your pelvic floor and bladder, you can become incontinent and even develop a prolapsed uterus. Doing kegels alone and creating a heroically strong pelvic floor won't hold all this together. You need to learn how to stop squeezing your pelvis and trunk like a tube of toothpaste as your support strategy, and start moving with your hips, legs, and abdominals. Good functional strength requires developing movement skill with a balance of stability and mobility. If you end up—consciously or subconsciously—choosing rigidity to stabilize an area of your body, you may develop strength but should be walking around with a sticker on your forehead that says "Warning: Contents Under Pressure, May Explode at Any Time."

Many women can't wait to return to the gym after pregnancy to work on toning up their stretched-out bodies. I would recommend treating the process as rehabilitation and not fitness, regardless if you had a vaginal or C-section birth; either way, muscles have been damaged and need a chance to recover. The time frame for soft tissue healing is four to six weeks, and most of that will happen in the first three weeks. However, you should still be cautious in weeks three to six, because even though you may be feeling better, your body is still trying to remodel tissues back to their strong and functional states.

WhyThingsHurt.com has a list of videos that you should watch in their particular order to learn about pain, posture, and movement. The first few videos will teach you what is "normal," and the rest will demonstrate exercises to help you restore normal movement. Start at the beginning and work down. Once you can complete these movements well, you should be ready to take what you have learned to the gym.

# Beth's Story: An Ex-Runner-Turned-Mother Rediscovers Her Body

Beth was an energetic nurse in her mid-thirties with two young boys to chase around. In her early twenties she was an elite runner, but these days walking a few blocks was a painful chore, and picking up her kids was nearly impossible. Pregnancy had done a number on Beth—twice. She had endured the slow nine months of body changes. She had powered through the labors and deliveries and ended up with two lovely little boys to watch grow and thrive, but her body, as a result, decided to stop cooperating with her desired lifestyle. She went from competitive running, to running a few times a week with discomfort, to chasing her kids around in pain, to walking being a painful task, all in a period of just a few years.

When Beth first walked into my office, she stated that she had tried physiotherapy, massage, chiropractic adjustments, core training, prolotherapy, and intramuscular stimulation (IMS) for her back problems, all with mixed success. IMS had provided her with the most relief, but she still sat in front of me with a dysfunctional body, so she obviously needed something more or different to help her get her body back. Her goals were simple: to walk without pain, play with her toddlers, and generally live an active lifestyle. I had to push her to include running on that list, because she, at the age of thirty-seven, had resigned herself to the idea that she would never run again.

To look at her, Beth was a thin, lean runner with a big smile and a positive attitude even though her body was failing her. She appeared to have all the pieces, so why was she having so much trouble? Therapists had massaged her, needled her, stretched her, cracked her, and strengthened her, but she still couldn't walk without significant discomfort in her back. The problem seemed to be that no one took the time to teach her how her body functions biomechanically. Loosening things and strengthen things were helpful, but she needed to understand the basic concepts of how to live in her body. The "why" and the "how" she needed to do things with her body became much more important than "what" she needed to do. I explained the why and the how to her, and once she started to gain control of her body and her symptoms, running began to look possible again.

Beth's biggest challenge was that she was relatively hypermobile, or loose-jointed, particularly in her hips. It becomes challenging, especially for a hypermobile new mom, to determine how to balance her upper body on her lower body; most people who haven't been through pregnancy have a difficult time standing, sitting and walking properly, so I am always impressed when some women bounce back after having a baby, and I am not surprised when many have trouble.

In order to effectively stack up your skeleton for functional movement, your ab muscles work together with your butt and the backs of your legs, while your back muscles pair together with your thighs. Life, sports, work, and genetics result in common variations of these pairings, and the resulting postural muscle imbalances can create pain over time. Pregnancy has to be the most common single biggest life event that will change a person's posture.

Beth's body slowly grew heavier over nine months. Her pelvis, hips, and feet became even looser due to hormonal changes. Her abdominals were slowly stretched out and her weight distribution changed as her belly enlarged. Her organs were slowly moving to new locations in her abdomen as the baby grew. After nine months of slow changes, Beth's labor created fast and dramatic body changes. She likely lost twenty pounds in one day, her stretched-out abs lost all their tension, her pelvic floor was damaged, and now she had to carry and care for a rapidly growing human twenty-four hours a day. To her credit, she got through that process twice, but after a few years, she needed a few key areas to be loosened in her body, and then to literally be taught how to stand, sit, walk, breathe, bend and lift again. She could do all those things, but her way hurt. I taught her how her body was built to do them, and how her way, although easier, was causing the problem.

Beth had a small diastasis (or separation/hernia) in her upper abdominals, just below her rib cage; this drew therapists to help her train her abs. Beth had mild urinary incontinence; this drew therapists to teach her pelvic-floor kegels. Beth had overly flexible hips; this drew therapists to give her leg-strengthening exercises. She had all the pieces addressed, but no one effectively taught her how to hold them together in a coordinated manner.

Looking into her past, Beth was a gymnast before she was a runner, and her posture showed it. She had "chest up, shoulders back and down" ingrained into her. She held herself up from her mid back, and when she moved or bent she kept her mid torso nice and braced. It wasn't surprising that the small hernia in the front of her torso was at the exact same level as where she holds all the tension in her back. When there was no room to move in her back, the tension and pressure of her abdomen had to go somewhere, so it bulged forward and inhibited her abdominal wall; that tear was a warning sign of bad torso posture but a red herring for her back pain.

The back dominant-muscle imbalance that Beth had developed in her torso made it difficult for her to effectively balance her upper body on her lower body. Overly bracing her mid back was tipping Beth's torso backward and levering her loosey-goosey hips and pelvis forward, causing compression in her lower back, SI (sacroiliac) joints, and hip sockets. It was this pattern of movement that was ultimately responsible for most of her pain. The pattern stemmed from the combination of a learned behavior in a childhood sport, her genetic hypermobility, and the effects of pregnancy and motherhood. The learned behavior is the only changeable aspect in that list, so that's what we worked on.

I explained this all to Beth while showing her in the mirror, and I walked her through the process of release, re-educate, rebuild. We would find and loosen the tight areas that were causing her problems, and then I would teach her how to stand, sit, and move differently; only when she could wrap her brain around how to physically perform her day-to-day tasks would we start extra strengthening exercises. She agreed, so we began the process with what she had already found to work—IMS.

Even though her hips had an incredible amount of flexibility, it was evident that the tension in her deep hip rotator muscles was part of her pain, so I needled her glutes, piriformis, tensor fascia lata, and their tug-of-war buddy, the adductor longus, in her groin. Beth felt better immediately, but I knew that I had only loosened the tension created by her compensation pattern, and that it would eventually return if she was left to her own devices; I therefore taught her about how she was holding her trunk. I showed her in the mirror her side profile, and helped her see what I was talking about, before sending her home with the project of thinking about her torso and to observe how other people hold themselves in funny ways.

**Relevant videos on WhyThingsHurt.com:**

- Everything Your Mother Taught You about Posture is WRONG
- How to Stand
- How to Sit
- 4-Point Neutral Spine

She came back to see me feeling better, with the suspicion that we were onto something. Although her back was still sore and her new posture seemed impossible to sustain for very long, she experienced less pain and felt stronger when she paid attention to her trunk, instead of the pain in her pelvis and back. Rather than trying to focus her on turning on her "core muscles," I demonstrated that if she puts her body in the right position, her core muscles will activate on their own—a practice that is more sustainable long term and the way your body is supposed to work.

Once Beth became more comfortable with standing and sitting tasks, she needed to learn how to move and not forget everything she had learned about staying still. Effective movement requires stabilization of some areas and dissociation of others. People with chronic pain tend to strongly brace particular areas, while moving in the joints that are left over; this practice helps prevent acute pain in the short term but produces chronic issues over time.

**The re-educate process I walked Beth through (videos on WhyThingsHurt.com):**

1. Beth needed to learn how to support her trunk in a neutral position and to then freely move in her hips.
    - 🎬 "4-Point Neutral Spine"
    - 🎬 "4-Point Rock-backs"

2. Beth needed to learn how to breathe into her rib cage and not brace her back.
    - 🎬 "How to Sit"
    - 🎬 "Breathing as an Exercise"
    - 🎬 "Rib Shimmy"

3. Beth needed to discover how to use her feet to support her hips.
    - 🎬 "Foot Tripod"
    - 🎬 "Foot Flex"
    - 🎬 "Ankle Skewer"
    - 🎬 "One-leg Stand"

4. Beth needed to understand that her chest tightness and forward-head posture were making her compensate and brace her torso backward.
    - 🎬 "Why Necks Hurt"
    - 🎬 "Why Mid Backs Hurt"

5. Beth needed to see that when she lifted her arms up in front of her, her entire torso leaned backward, but with awareness and practice, she learned to control it.
    - 🎬 "Why Shoulders Hurt"
    - 🎬 "Reaching Up 11"
    - 🎬 "Air Bench Press"

I only treated Beth once with IMS before teaching her movement. Each week she came back with a new "Aha!" sensation about her body and a revelation that she needed to be more careful about how much she does in a day or a week. She suffered a few setbacks and flare ups that required IMS, but since she was learning to control her body, she knew when she needed a tune-up, and she would bounce back faster instead of going into a pain cycle every few weeks. She started moving better and better, so I gave more difficult exercises to perform:

1. I taught her how to use her legs while stabilizing her torso.
    - 🎬 "Kneeling Squats"

2. I taught her how to use her hips, knees, ankles and feet while stabilizing her torso.

- 🎬 "Squats"
- 🎬 "Thirsty Birds"

3. I taught her how to move sideways.

- 🎬 "Speed Skater"
- 🎬 "Half-Squat Crab Walk"

Although she was moving better and feeling better, she kept complaining that the pain in her left SI joint wouldn't go away. Initially with Beth, I got the sense that if I released anything on her, it would only return because of her movement habits, but now that she moved better and continued to experience a specific pain, I felt it was my turn to work on her again. This time, I assessed her visceral system in more detail by manually assessing the fascial mobility of the organs in her abdomen and pelvis. What I found was a restriction in her sigmoid colon and in some of the loops of her small intestine. The sigmoid colon sits just on the inside of the left SI joint and can cause persistent left SI pain and even sciatica. I performed visceral manipulation with her to free the left side of her pelvis from the front and let her go with the confidence that she was moving better. The result was that she canceled her follow-up appointment, because she was feeling so good and was now able to physically play with her kids.

Beth's path to improvement was not a linear one. She had her flare ups, but we continued to push the envelope of what she could do. We introduced jumping, pushing, pulling and twisting, with a strong focus on form and function. She is now aware of her body with daily movements, she can walk and play with her kids with little-to-no pain, and she is able to start a walk-run program to rebuild her fitness. She comes in for semi-regular tune-ups of IMS, exercise progression, and the occasional visceral work, but she is largely independent and living the active lifestyle she couldn't previously manage.

Beth's story is an extremely common one for women after pregnancy. As a physiotherapist, I can see the effects of pregnancy on women's movement and posture even decades later. I find that with a little help and direction, most women can find their way out of the physical turmoil that results from pregnancy. IMS, movement training, and visceral work tend to be the three missing ingredients.

# How to Stand

It may seem like an odd concept to relearn how to do something that you first learned as a baby, but trust me: there are more nuances to standing properly than you likely appreciate. You have grown since you were one, hurt yourself, become stressed out, sat at a desk for years, grew self-conscious, and now you wonder why your back hurts sometimes for no particular reason. To a physiotherapist like me, how you stand is a reflection of who you are. There is a story in everyone's body, and if you understand your own, you can dramatically improve your future physical health.

Gravity is a constant, unrelenting force that is trying to flatten you into the ground, and it is your job to use your brain and your muscles to help your skeleton hold your body up in a functionally vertical position. Just because you can stand doesn't mean that you do it very well, so I will give you some tips on what to pay attention to in order to improve your standing posture.

Start by stripping down to your underwear and look at your front and side profiles in the mirror. Try to get a general sense of where you hold most of your tension, and see if it resembles any of the below illustrations:

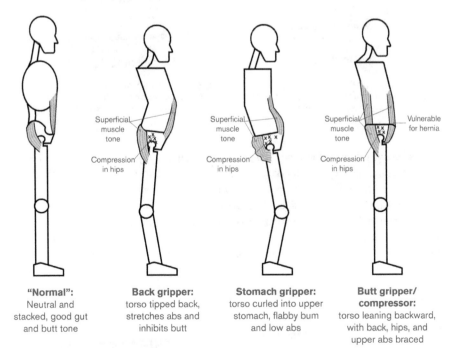

**"Normal":**
Neutral and stacked, good gut and butt tone

**Back gripper:**
torso tipped back, stretches abs and inhibits butt

**Stomach gripper:**
torso curled into upper stomach, flabby bum and low abs

**Butt gripper/ compressor:**
torso leaning backward, with back, hips, and upper abs braced

Is your torso tipped backward? Do your knees overly straighten? Is your butt tucked under or sticking out? Is all your weight on your heels? Try to gauge which posture type you are, or ask someone to take a picture of your back—you may be surprised at the results.

No matter which picture you look like, start by taking a deep breath. Where did all the air go? Did your shoulders shrug up to your ears? Did your rib cage open laterally? Did your belly distend down? To improve your posture, the first area to pay attention to is around your diaphragm, or just below the bra strap area. Your torso is the longest part of your spine and contains the most joints, so it is the best starting point. The objective of standing up tall is to vertically elongate your torso like you are pulling on either end of a slinky. The ribs should spread apart and lift the head and shoulders up while lifting pressure off of the abdomen. The greatest mistake in this area is to put too much focus on lifting up the chest and pinning down the shoulders, because while that opens up the front of your slinky, it compresses all the rings around the back.

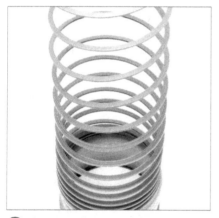

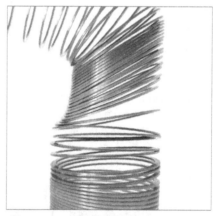

 Standing up tall should be like pulling on either end of a slinky, elongating the torso and taking pressure off the abdomen.

Standing up tall should not put too much focus on lifting up the chest and pinning down the shoulders, because you will be compressing all the rings around the back.

It is beneficial to understand the differences between moving your shoulders back and forth, versus slouching, or extending your upper back, because they are two different movements. For optimal standing posture, you want to use your rib cage to support your shoulders, not your shoulders to support your rib cage. You should be able to feel the internal lifting, lateral support from your diaphragm without tipping your entire torso backward. Imagine that your ribs are the rings of the slinky and that you are lengthening all the way around, and not just the front. Lifting only the front will inhibit your abdominals from working properly and compress your back.

Trying to control all the moving parts of your body is like being given two buttons and told to push them both in, but you are only allowed to use one finger, and one pops back out every time you push the other. Correcting one area of your body will likely alter the position of another area, either positively or negatively, so you need to understand which areas require attention. Opening up the back of your rib cage may feel as though you are leaning forward or it may shift all your weight back onto your heels. Look at your side profile in a mirror to help understand what you may not yet feel.

Your body has many moving parts, and each one is sending feedback to your brain as to where it is in space, which is helpful but can also make changing long-standing postural habits more challenging. Your brain has a head-righting reflex that wants to keep your face and eyes looking straight forward, and it will tend to have your body accommodate your neck to achieve an easier visual field. When you shift your attention to lengthening your lower torso instead of subconsciously compensating for your eyes, you may realize that you have either a head-forward posture or tend to overly retract your head backward, resulting in a flat neck; this is when a mirror comes in handy to see where your head is in relation to your body. Try not to control your posture from your head, but instead build a better pedestal for it to sit by focusing on your trunk. Avoid the temptation to retract your head, and instead work on lengthening your "slinky" in order for your head to sit on top of your trunk.

Your pelvis and hips are the center of your universe. They are where your upper body connects to your lower body and where everything goes wrong posturally. While standing, the pelvic area can shift forward and backward in space, and it can tip anteriorly or posteriorly on your hip sockets. Your hips can also rotate inward or outward in the sockets, which will affect how you load weight on your feet. This is the major crossroad of the body, and it is worth understanding, even superficially.

The objective in standing well is to vertically stack all of the joints in your spine, pelvis, hips, knees, ankles, and feet in a strong and functional position. Your pelvis should balance on your hips in a slight forward tilt and be situated underneath your trunk and over-top of your knees. It may sound obvious, but you will notice that some people hold their pelvis well in front of their trunk and tucked under them, while others hold their pelvis well behind their trunk with a big swayback. Strive to vertically stack your body parts to achieve a gentle S-curve in your spine.

When a "bum tucker" draws back their pelvis beneath their torso and over their knees, they may see just how much their head is poking forward; conversely, when a "swaybacker" pushes their pelvis forward and under, they may notice that their torso wants to lean backward. Creating this awareness in a mirror is an important step to controlling and improving your posture. It can be frustrating, but I promise that it is a useful exercise. Some people, when they start paying attention, will realize that they are subconsciously clenching their butt while standing, and others will literally have no concept of how to contract their butt muscles. When I start teaching clients, I encourage them to improve their posture by asking themselves ten times a day, "What am I doing with my butt right now?" It goes a long way in creating basic awareness of how their hips are sitting in their sockets and how their hips relate to their pelvis.

You will find that if you try to subtly rotate your upper thighs inward or outward while standing, it will alter the position of your sits bones (the two bones in your butt that you sit on) in the back of your pelvis, as well as how you load weight onto your feet. Bum tuckers tend to hold their sits bones compressed together and will find that gently rotating their upper thighs inward will open up the back of their pelvis and help them to properly use the muscles on the sides of their hips. No matter your current postural pattern, it is helpful to realize that your hips can rest in their sockets in different ways based on your muscle tension. If you learn to appreciate the fact that you can influence how they sit, you can then begin to more assertively improve your standing posture.

Some people have really high arches with a stiff midfoot, while others have a more neutral foot and tend to pronate or collapse through their long arch. There is a major genetic component to your type of feet, but you also play a significant role in either maintaining or destroying your feet; unfortunately, it is commonly the latter. (For more of my views on orthotics and shoes, please refer to Section 4, "Shoes: Good Support or Coffins for Your Feet?") The type of shoes you choose to wear will significantly impact your posture. If you are serious about improving your posture, one of the best things you can do is to spend more time barefoot or in minimalist shoes that allow your body to receive feedback from your feet about how they are interacting with the ground. We tend to overly cushion our shoes and elevate the heels, which throws off our body's perception of where we are in space, typically making us overcompensate in our calf and hip muscles.

To improve your posture, think of your feet as tripods, with weight on the heels and the balls of your feet. Your toes should also be able to actively spread and press down into the ground. Looking at your side profile in the mirror, imagine your feet are cemented to the ground and skewered through your ankles; practice leaning forward through this skewer to load weight on the front of your feet. We do not typically load the middle or front of our feet efficiently because of our shoes, and, in turn, we lose touch with how to bring our shins forward over our feet—a task that is required to walk and run properly. How well the arches of your feet are maintained is largely a by-product of the muscle balance in your hips, calves and feet.

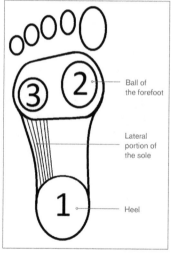

Foot should bear weight like a tripod and have lengthwise tension for support.

Freeing up the tension in these areas with IMS (intramuscular stimulation), followed by teaching a person about the ankle skewer and hip rotations, can retrain and strengthen most feet—as long as the person is willing to work at it. Your arches won't collapse if you learn to stand properly, but there are both trickle-up and trickle-down effects on the feet, so you must be willing to address your entire body.

Finally, consider your head and shoulders. Most people focus only on these two body parts, but I believe they should be the last areas to address. Your shoulders are intimately connected to both your trunk and your neck by means of your pecs, upper traps, and lats. We tend to become tight in all of these muscle groups due to work, life and sports, and they have an impact on our posture. If you take my advice and work first on correcting your trunk posture, you may find that your shoulders now feel hunched forward and you want to pull them back. Your trunk has likely overcompensated for the tightness in your chest and shoulders, and now you need to deal with these short muscles. If you first understand how to control your trunk, you will be able lengthen your shoulder muscles much more effectively.

While standing, lightly attempt to draw your two shoulders away from each other, and support them from underneath with your ribs instead of pinching your shoulder blades together. Avoid retracting your head and instead focus on lifting the very top of your slinky—your head will rise if you lift your upper ribs.

I know this is too many things to think about all at once while standing, but if you break the above advice into parts and build body awareness through movement, it will become clearer. A series of basic exercise videos to help walk you through the steps are available on WhyThingsHurt.com.

# How to Sit

Who taught you how to sit? I'm guessing nobody. You likely figured it out by trial and error while you were a baby. You learned how to stay upright, and eventually not fall over, while resting on your butt; that was a major milestone when you were eight months old, but you haven't been given much credit for it later in life, have you? Unfortunately, it's later on when you will need to be good at it, because chances are you're going to be spending multiple hours a day staring at a computer screen. It is time you learned how to sit properly.

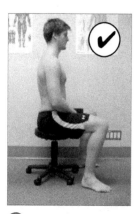 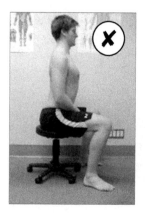 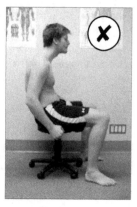

 Good sitting and bad sitting postures. Sitting properly is a skill that should be learned.

Our bodies are built to deal with the vertical load of gravity, but at the same time they are inherently lazy when it comes to holding up everything properly. We have a tendency to become engrossed in what is visually in front of us, with little regard to how we have positioned our bodies to allow our eyes to see what we want to see. Your brain has a head-righting reflex that tries to keep your head looking straight forward in the easiest way possible; unfortunately, this usually comes at the expense of your neck and back.

The goal of sitting properly is to vertically stack your torso and head on top of your pelvis and hips in a gentle S-curve. The odds of you doing this properly are unlikely for a few reasons. First, most people experience one, two, or three of the following: a forward-head posture, an overly braced lower torso, and/or very flexible or stiff hips.

Second, most chairs are not designed ergonomically and promote slouching more than support. Finally, life tends to get in the way of your awareness of gravity and proper posture, and you sit the way your body takes you. If you create some body awareness, learn how to use your chair properly, and have someone help you with your physical restrictions, sitting properly can significantly diminish the chronic tension and pain that can come from working a long day at a desk.

Begin by learning how to situate your pelvis on top of your hips, not behind or in front of them. Some people sit on their tailbone, while others tend to sit on their upper legs. It requires a balance of your hip flexors, abdominals, and back muscles to stack everything, and have you sit on your sits bones properly (these are the deep bones in your butt). The sits bones should be back on the chair and spread wide apart to create a stable base, not tucked underneath you and together. This position of your pelvis is most important, because it sets the foundation of the natural S-curve of your spine.

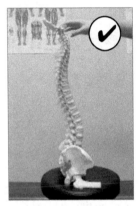
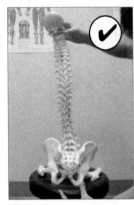
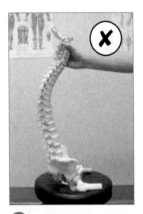

 Good stacking.　　 Sits bones apart.　　 Pelvis behind hips.

When your pelvis is rolled backward and your sits bones are together, your back muscles will have to work harder to sit up straight. Therefore, step one is get your butt underneath you!

Step two is to situate your torso over-top of your pelvis without lurching it forward, leaning it backward, or slouching it downward. Those who sit on their tailbones will have a tendency to let their entire body collapse into a slouch, while those who sit on their upper legs tend to perch on the edge of the chair and hold their torso in front of their hips. The most hypermobile of people tend to do both; they will perch on the edge until they get tired then collapse into a slouch. Stiff people, meanwhile, will immediately start with their hips in front, lean back their torso and push their heads forward. We all have our own strategies, but the one position that allows us to sit efficiently is the one that stacks the spine and allows the skeleton to do most of the work, instead of the muscles and ligaments.

Creating awareness of their torso position is often difficult for people, because they rarely think about what their mid and lower back is doing. Learning to not overly brace your back, and instead use your diaphragm and abs for support, are important lessons to help you sit well. Use a mirror and look at your side profile to try and create a vertical line down the midline of your torso through your hip socket. You will likely find that your torso either wants to be tipped forward or tipped backward, and that if you achieve straightness, your head might be pushed well forward; here is where you learn how much your trunk and pelvis have been accommodating your neck.

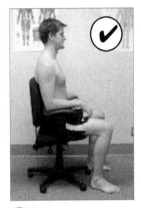 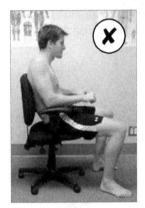 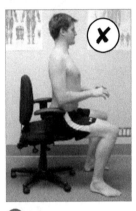

 Well stacked.   Butt and head forward.   Don't perch!

Your upper back is relatively the stiffest part of your spine, and if it becomes rounded, it will push your head forward. Your body will compensate for this by tipping your head up and chin forward by extending your lower torso, or by sliding your butt forward on the chair in attempt to place your body beneath your head in the easiest possible way. These practices are immediately the most comfortable when you sit, but they are the exact positions that lead to pain and your posture worsening over time.

Your upper back doesn't move much, so when you try to lift your head and chest, it should be a subtle, gentle movement that elongates your upper spine, instead of leaning you backward. It should be a movement that doesn't negatively alter the positions you have found with your torso and pelvis below. When you effectively position your pelvis on your hips, your torso on your pelvis, and your head on your torso, it will look great but might feel challenging to hold. The muscles you feel working are the ones you need to strengthen, and just sitting properly can help do this. People who tend to sit back on their tailbones will have to learn to use their hip flexors and low abs to hold the pelvis forward over the hips. People who sit on their upper legs have to learn to release their back and draw their rib cage backward over their hips, using their back together with their abs instead of in place of. Many people have to learn to do both.

Your hip flexors attach the front of your lower spine and the inside bowl part of your pelvis down into your groin. To use them effectively for sitting, it will feel as though you are using your lower stomach muscles. Once you have shimmied your butt underneath you, try to gently pull your pubic bone down to the floor. This should create a tension in your lower stomach and act to slightly tip your pelvis over-top of your hips; if this forces your torso forward, then you are using your back muscles and not your hip flexors. If your lower torso is forward, place your two hands on your lower rib cage and try to gently slouch it backward, all while maintaining your hip flexors. The tendency

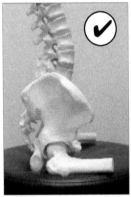
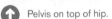
⬆ Pelvis on top of hip.

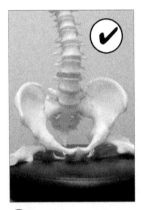

⬆ Front view.

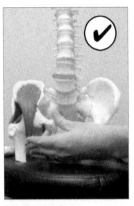
⬆ Hip flexor holds pelvis forward.

is to do too much or nothing at all—a deep C-curve instead of a gentle S-curve. You must hold your pelvis forward and your rib cage back. You will find that the video on WhyThingsHurt.com called "How to Sit" demonstrates these concepts well.

Chairs can either help or hinder your efforts to sit well. If you are tall or short, chairs are likely not made to support your frame, so learning how to use them is that much more important. Ideally, a chair is high enough that your knees end up slightly below your hips, or a hip angle of about 90 degrees. It should also be short enough that your feet rest flat on the floor and that you can sit back against the backrest without the seat pan pressing into your upper calves. If your thighs are quite short, you should buy a smaller chair or place an additional back support behind you on the backrest. On adjustable desk chairs, there are typically two levers on the side: one adjusts the height of the chair and the other affects the angle of the seat pan and the backrest. You want the backrest angled forward enough that when you sit back, it supports your torso in a position that is relatively over top of your hips, not well behind it.

If you have a significant head-forward posture, sitting with your torso more vertical will feel like you are leaning forward, but it is only your head that is in front of you; use a mirror to see what you feel, and reality might reveal two different things. Your body will naturally slide your hips forward on the chair and want your torso to lean backward to accommodate your head; don't allow it. Keep your butt underneath you, with your torso supported vertically by the chair, and focus on elongating your neck and head upward, not backward.

If you set up your chair well, it will allow the lumbar support and the backrest to support your torso so that sitting becomes a relatively passive process for your back. Sitting poorly for eight hours a day can be harder on your body than a contact sport, so learn to sit back in your chair and let it do most of the work. Your job is simply to maintain some awareness of gravity and to reposition yourself every fifteen minutes or so.

# How to Walk

People watching is one of my favorite pastimes, because I appreciate the story in everyone. I loved it when a large black woman, confidently strutting down the Vegas strip, sassily told my buddy (who was wearing silk, leopard-print pajamas during his bachelor party) that he "looked like her bedspread." I am amazed by the seventy-five-year-old, tanned leathery old man who wears nothing but a glorified loin cloth when hiking up and down the beach in Hawaii when I see him every Christmas. I am curious about the homeless guy I see limping down the back alley near my office every week, and I am fascinated by watching my children discover everything for the first time. Everyone has a story, and everyone moves in their own way as a result. I try not to interfere with anyone's story, but instead provide the guidance to help a person take their story down a better future path if they are ready to listen. Improving how you walk is a difficult task but a doable one, so long as you are willing to pay attention to yourself and not let frustration stop you.

Everything you may have learned in the previous sections about sitting and standing is relevant to how you walk. Your walking style is a projection of both your confidence and your physical well-being. It's a subconscious act for the majority of your life, but it takes a lot of concentration at the beginning and end, when getting your body to cooperate with you can be an all-consuming task. Babies try their best to gain control over their spinal reflexes to coordinate their legs and to stay upright, while aging seniors try their best to overcome the stiffness and weakness that has made balance an ever-growing challenge. The large cohort of healthy, mobile people in-between these two stages is rarely forced to think about how they walk, because their brain and spinal cord seem to do it for them. The body moves on autopilot by creating what are called motor programs, so that you don't have to think about every little movement that happens as you walk and run. These motor programs free your brain to attend to other aspects of your environment as you move around, but what happens when your autopilot isn't the best driver in the world?

Your motor programs are developed by movement experience over the years, and develop compensations based on factors like shoes and injuries, but they are also influenced by mental aspects such as self-confidence. The way you walk becomes a reflection of who you are, and has the capacity to slowly but surely create long-standing physical problems if not done well. If you suffer from chronic pain and haven't been able to find lasting relief in any form of treatment, then it is entirely possible that you need to change some of your fundamental habits such as how you walk. Start by paying attention to how differently everyone else walks. It is easier to begin by projecting your attention outward to provide a better context before you focus your awareness inward.

The goal of walking is usually to get from point A to point B. Sometimes the path is flat, sometimes it is bumpy, or it might be uphill or downhill. Your body is equipped to deal with most terrain, but to start, we will assume that you are walking on flat, level ground. It is your lower body's job to do most of the work, but it is your upper body that tends to cause problems, because it contains more movable hinges. Imagine that I gave you three blocks and asked you to stack them on top of each other and quickly walk across the room; it would take some concentration, but it wouldn't be too challenging. Now imagine I gave you twelve more blocks; the lever just grew longer and the task became much trickier. The posture of your torso is the long lever that can make walking properly difficult. You may recall the illustrations in Section I, "Why Hips Hurt," which demonstrate the role of some major hinges in the body. Look at the pictures below and consider the impact that each of these various hinges and postures may have on the body when your legs are creating a torque from the bottom while trying to walk:

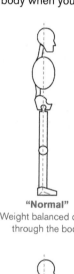 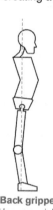 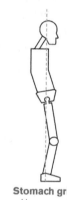 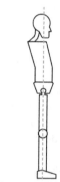

| **"Normal"** | **Back gripper** | **Stomach gripper** | **Butt and back gripper** |
|---|---|---|---|
| Weight balanced down through the body | Uneven weight distribution | Uneven weight distribution | Weight shifted to back line of body |

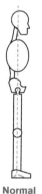 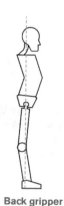 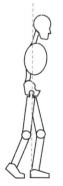 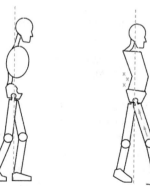

| **Normal standing** | **Back gripper standing** | **Normal walking** | **Back gripper walking** |
|---|---|---|---|
| | | Slight forward lean from ankle and weight over foot at impact | Increased heel impact and weight behind foot at impact, creating a jarring force with every step |

When you walk forward, your lower body is charged with the task of staying beneath your upper body well enough so that you don't fall down, but your upper body quite often leans backward even though you want to go forward. I liken this phenomenon to driving with your emergency brake on, because your deep hip muscles have to work overtime to prevent your tower from tumbling. When your torso posture is far enough from the norm, either braced backward or slouched forward, it inhibits your gluteus maximus (the bigger muscle of your butt) from doing its job of pushing you forward properly, and as a result, your walking gait will be compromised.

People who are braced in their upper back tend to pull the top of their tower backward, which results in them taking long strides out in front of them, with their heel striking the ground, creating an impact-breaking force with every step. On the other hand, people who hold their torsos slouched forward with their bums tucked beneath tend to take shorter steps and impact on a flat foot, merely pulling themselves along. Neither of these strategies will result in the person actually using their butt to propel them forward, and both tend to result in pain issues in the back, hips, knees or shins over time.

To walk properly, you must first gain some awareness of your torso posture and work at holding it in a tall, lengthened position, with your shoulders relaxed and your arms hanging freely. Your first movement should be a subtle forward lean from your ankle, paired with the gentle contraction of your abdominals. Your abdominals create a muscular wall that attaches the front of your rib cage to the front of your pelvis, which can prevent your torso from hinging backward as the torque from your leg propels you forward. Your butt and hamstring should contract to pull your leg backward, which should be matched by a gentle bracing in your abdominals and an engagement of your foot to grab the ground in order to create the torque to push you forward. Unfortunately, the biomechanics of this movement are commonly compromised by shoes and postural imbalances. If you are having trouble getting your glutes to fire, start working on opening up your mid back and learn how to load your shin over-top of your foot more effectively.

To help people understand the role of their ankles, I compare them to the two-wheeled Segway scooters: in order to move forward, you have to lean your center of gravity forward; the further you lean, the faster you go. To stop, you balance your center of gravity over the two wheels, and to back up, you lean your weight slightly behind your base of support. Similarly, in order to walk well, you need to use your ankles, because they are important hinges that drive your gait. Think of your body as a long plank with a hinge at your ankle, leaning slightly forward so that your sternum is just ahead of your pelvis. This will help keep your stride short so that your foot hits the ground underneath you instead of ahead of you. It will also help to make your foot strike become more about weight transfer and less about impact, because your legs will have to move quickly to keep up with your tower that is leaning forward. You would likely do the same thing if you tried to carry a stack of blocks quickly across the room; a slight forward lean in the tower will help the blocks not fall off the back as you move.

Paying attention to where in your body you are actually leaning can be a tricky task due to your brain's perception of what feels normal, as well as the various tightness and weakness throughout your body. Some people have significant forward-head posture, while others have braced mid backs or knees that hyperextend, but no matter where your imbalance is, your body has created a hangout place that your brain thinks is "normal." Anything that strays from this perceived "normal" is going to feel unnatural. Use a mirror to look at your side profile, and try to hold yourself in your best standing posture based on my discussions in the previous sections. Now, imagine that I cemented your feet to the floor and skewered you through your ankles; try to stay tall through your body, and practice leaning forward from your ankle hinges to feel the front of your feet engage the floor. Feel the difference between bending forward at your hip versus bringing your shins forward over your feet along with the rest of your body.

Most people who come into my office complain that their hip flexors are too tight but never understand why. My explanation typically starts from how they are holding their torso, helping them understand the pulls of their different hip flexor muscles. I find that the more braced or tipped backward someone is in their mid back, the more overworked and tight their big, superficial hip flexors become trying to counterbalance their pelvis and hip with their torso posture. This superficial hip flexor is called the tensor fasciae lata (TFL), and too much tension in it will effectively draw the hip forward in the socket, tighten up the IT band, and limit the proper hip extension required to walk and run efficiently. At the same time, the deeper hip flexor muscles (the iliacus and psoas) don't properly fire, and become ineffective at stabilizing the hip deep in its socket, resulting in hip, pelvis, knee and back pain. If you want a longer-term solution for your hip flexor tightness than foam rolling your TFLs every other day, try working on your torso posture and figure out how to use and strengthen your psoas.

When you are walking, you should hold yourself tall from your diaphragm, lean forward from your ankles, and look toward the horizon—not at the ground three feet in front of you. You should feel that your hamstrings and butt are pushing you forward as your hip extends behind you and as your TFL stretches. Your weight should transfer from the outside of your foot at impact toward your big toe as your foot leaves the ground. Your shoulders should hang and swing in a relaxed fashion at your sides as they are being held up by your rib cage—not braced back and together. Your feet and toes should engage the ground through your shoe, and your abdominals should be gently engaged. Finally, you should breathe and relax, trying to enjoy your surroundings, because although it may feel awkward to change your gait, you likely don't look as strange as you feel, and no one else really cares.

Visit WhyThingsHurt.com for videos to help you improve your hip, pelvis and torso awareness in order to improve your gait.

# Breathing: More Than Just Keeping You Alive

There are many systems that function subconsciously in your body that you likely take for granted, and rarely, if ever, think about. Among the most important of these is breathing. Breathing is an amazing physiological process that allows you to draw oxygen from the air around you and filter it into your blood stream to keep you alive. Your brain and spinal cord automatically do this for you. You breathe faster when you run, and slower when you sleep; your body determines how much oxygen you need and alters your breathing rate accordingly. The drawback of not being an active participant in your breathing pattern is that you can lose touch with what is "normal" for your body and be unaware of how things like pain, stress and posture are affecting you.

A basic understanding of the biomechanics of breathing and posture will help you understand what I mean. Your rib cage and thoracic spine are the structural foundation of your torso. Its rigidity protects your organs and supports your shoulders and neck, while its mobility helps you breathe, twist and move. Your lungs line the inside of your rib cage. In order for you to draw air into them, your rib cage needs to expand slightly and your diaphragm needs to contract and pull down; this creates a negative pressure and air is pulled inward. The elastic recoil of your rib cage and diaphragm passively push the air out to complete the breathing cycle. This keeps you alive.

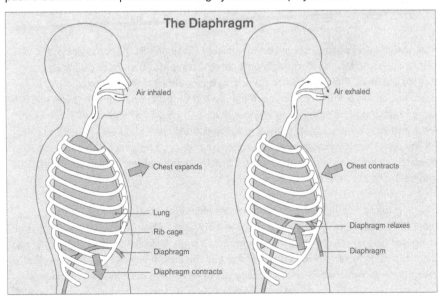

The diaphragm is comprised of two big muscular domes inside your lower trunk. Imagine opening a small umbrella inside your rib cage.

There is, obviously, a difference between being alive and breathing well. Just because you can breathe doesn't mean that you are doing it well. There is a connection between how you breathe and how you stand, largely due to the role of your diaphragm and the muscles in your mid to lower back. Your diaphragm is a big muscular dome that connects and supports the lower part of your rib cage. It is an integral part of breathing, but it also plays a major role in supporting your torso vertically from the inside. Poor use of the diaphragm, among other muscles, leads to the torso tipping backward when you attempt to stand up straight. The result is compression and immobility of the lower-back half of the rib cage. Unfortunately, this is what most people do when cued to lift their chest up and pull their shoulders back and down. It opens the front of the rib cage but closes down the back, resulting in a chronic tension in the back, shoulders and neck—not to mention a restricted lung capacity, because the rib cage won't expand very well.

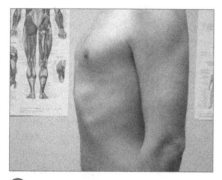

Poor diaphragm use: tipped backward.

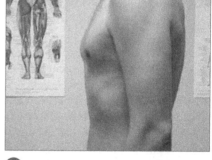

Good diaphragm use: vertically stacked.

The goal of good posture should be to vertically lengthen and stack the spine and ribs, but most people tend to lengthen their front and compress their back during day-to-day life postures, then work on compressing their front by doing sit ups and plank exercises during a workout. The result can be a strong, immobile, stiff rib cage that will force breathing to be either quite shallow or all in the belly and shoulders. If you go for a run and your breathing rate rises, you will notice that your shoulders lift up and down as you pant to catch your breath. The stiffer your rib cage becomes, the more you will need to use these accessory muscles for breathing, even at rest, which can translate into neck and shoulder problems.

Learning to use the internal support structure of your diaphragm can be difficult, as most people are tight in their mid and lower-back area, which will inhibit the dome from lifting and opening the lower-back part of the rib cage. It is best to start with what I call the "rib shimmy" exercise to build awareness of the area. It will also help to have the area needled, manipulated, and or massaged to loosen the back muscles and joints.

Begin by sitting down and looking at your side profile in the mirror. If you have a significant forward-head posture, the lower part of your rib cage will be the part of your back that will accommodate your neck; it is easier to sway the lower back forward to lift your head than to actually lift your chest and head. Drawing your lower rib cage back may feel like you are leaning too far forward; this is when a mirror is useful to view your side profile. Your body may be straight with only your head pushing forward. Try to maintain your lower trunk position and attempt to lift your chest.

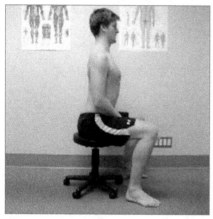

⬆ Overly braced rib cage.

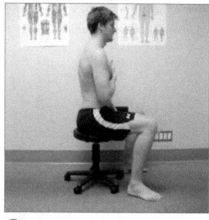

⬆ Good diaphragm support.

Breathing effectively with your diaphragm should expand your rib cage laterally (side to side) and posteriorly (from behind) to broaden your torso; it should not involve your shoulders lifting up to your ears. As you take a deep breath, you should feel your torso lengthen and lift as your ribs pull apart, but this should not make you tip backward. Learning to use this muscle further with occasional deep breaths will keep your torso more flexible. Using it to maintain the natural S-curve of your spine during exercise will help you engage your abdominals and protect your back, neck, and shoulders.

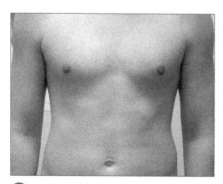

⬆ Before breath

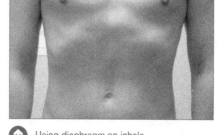

⬆ Using diaphragm on inhale

Pain, stress, emotion, and attitude will affect how you breathe and how you hold yourself physically. Stress and pain tend to make people tense and breathe shallowly, leading to further stiffness and more pain. Being either self-conscious or cocky is reflected in your physical posture, which can end up creating physical restrictions of proper breathing that can also lead to pain. Taking a few extra minutes to pay attention to how you breathe, sit, and stand can result in significantly improving your posture and reducing your pain. Learning to integrate the role of your diaphragm into your movement patterns will help you prevent injuries and maintain good posture.

Watch the "Breathing as an Exercise" video on WhyThingsHurt.com to further understand this section.

# Perseverance: Converting Challenge into Wisdom

In a span of less than two years leading up to publishing this book, I have undergone seven eye surgeries and am still functionally blind in my dominant eye. I have had two close family members be diagnosed with cancer, another die of ALS at age twenty-seven, and a third lose her baby well into her second trimester. I have had one close friend hospitalized for the better part of a year with acute pancreatitis, and a second with chronically collapsing lungs due to cystic fibrosis. In addition, some close family members who, while healthy, are going through major financial troubles, which have a ripple effect to the rest of the family. I have earned my badge in perseverance through it all, and I would like to share the wisdom I have developed along the way.

In the time between my fourth and fifth eye surgeries, when I had returned to work, I created an exercise in perspective for myself. In the same week, I visited my cousin Sam in the ICU, who had decided to stop life support in the coming months, I visited my friend Brian, who had undergone seven abdominal surgeries, and I visited Todd, who was sitting in his hospital bed with a chest tube inserted for three months waiting for his lung to hold. I was feeling down about my own health situation, but my friends helped me to see that things could always be worse, and that moping around was not going to help. Misery loves company, so we all supported each other the best we could. I happened to be the most functional of the downtrodden group, so I made the rounds.

Twenty-seven-year-old Sam was the one to teach me about the creation of wisdom just by how gracefully he handled his own situation. He was my wife's cousin who I superficially knew from the time he was about fourteen, but I got to know him quite well in his final year. He started having troubles with ALS-type symptoms and was diagnosed in the months surrounding my eye injury when I was in the midst of my deterioration, pain and three months of being bedridden. We connected with each other over Facebook, and with our worlds suddenly flipped upside down, we felt like we had each other when everything else seemed to be falling apart. Thankfully, I turned a corner and became functional again, but sadly Sam continued to worsen every month, but he remained supportive, empathetic, and positive until his final days. I visited him in the ICU a few times, and although he could only communicate by typing on his iPad, he inspired me to enjoy every moment and taught me the importance of controlling your own destiny. He connected with his family and friends in a new way, he explored religion, created bucket lists, got angry, shared laughs, and learned to stop and smell the roses, all while he couldn't have physically been in a worse predicament. When his body was progressively failing, but while he still possessed the ability to communicate his wishes, he decided to stop his life support on his own terms—a decision that couldn't make him any braver in my eyes.

Acceptance and control are the two keys that I believe allow us to find happiness, even in the face of adversity. They can be difficult to locate when things are going badly, but I saw Sam find peace of mind on the way out once he found a way to have both acceptance and control. My timeline for acceptance has been longer than Sam was given to process his life, but I have found that the more I am able come to terms with the fact that my eye and my vision aren't going to get any better, the happier I can be. I have to accept that I can't play some of the sports I love, and move forward to focus on what I can by taking control and actively making decisions to allow life to happen.

At work, I see many people who have been injured, where the greatest barrier holding them back from recovering is their inability to accept their current situation. Even though the injury wasn't their fault, they are responsible for dealing with it before they can move forward. Lack of acceptance tends to create a perceived lack of control, which can be a slippery slope to depression. I felt depression for the first time during my journey, and I still do from time to time, but I have chosen to consciously create wisdom from my challenges to find happiness again.

My friend Brian has always been a "foodie" and the one to introduce our group to new and interesting beers. We would have boys' weekends, and he would cater them for us with amazing food creations and beer pairings that would continue to blow us away. Unfortunately, he developed digestive problems over a period of years and progressively had to give up much of the food and beers that he brought into our lives and had centered his around. In early 2015, he became acutely ill and was rushed to hospital, where he was eventually diagnosed with acute pancreatitis. He was in and out of the ICU for months and faced surgery after surgery, the whole time being fed through a tube directly to his stomach. He didn't eat real food for six months! I had sports taken away from me, and he lost the ability to eat. When I visited him in the later part of his hospital sentence, he wasn't watching movies; he was looking up recipes on the Food Network. He focused on what he was going to do when he was better, and he didn't wallow in the unfortunate place he found himself.

Brian impressed me with his stoic acceptance and positive attitude while he was still in the thick of his hospital stay and medical procedures. I'm sure he was depressed and in pain for large portions of his nearly year-long stay in the hospital, but he appeared to have the emotional intelligence to take it in stride and not let the experience beat him. His demonstration of stoicism provided me with the motivation to get on with my life and not let my countless eye doctor appointments and surgeries interfere with my emotional well-being.

My five friends and I had partial season tickets to the Vancouver Canucks hockey games, but we were a banged up bunch that year. The third man down was Todd. Unlike Brian and I, Todd had dealt with a chronic condition his entire life: cystic fibrosis.

I wrecked my eye, Brian's guts didn't work, and Todd's lungs wouldn't cooperate. His chronic condition became acute that year when portions of his lungs kept collapsing. Hospitals had long since been a part of Todd's life, and regular exercise was his weapon to combat his chronic condition. This time, however, he was isolated from his twin daughters and could only lie around and do nothing for three months, waiting for his body to figure itself out—a helpless place to be.

While I was playing sports throughout my invincible years, Todd was gaining perspective on our healthcare system. Todd helped me to be more objective about my situation and to see life more as a journey rather than a terrible circumstance, because he had endured health challenges for over thirty years while continuing to maintain a positive attitude.

We all pay our dues at one time or another, and, unfortunately, some people are forced to endure much more than others. These challenges are where character is developed, and I have tried my best to learn something from every experience in my life as well as those of my friends, both good and bad.

While I was lying face down for a week after my fourth eye surgery, I stumbled upon Ryan Holiday's audiobook, The Obstacle is the Way, and received a history lesson in stoicism while I was living through my greatest obstacle in life to date. Ryan's book, combined with Tim Ferriss' blog, kept my stoic mind going and my entrepreneurial spirit alive while the world seemed far away. Writing this book has been an educational and cathartic experience for me, and one which Tim and Ryan have unknowingly helped to inspire. I had worked away on it for years before my accident, but having my world flipped upside down gave me the motivation to more assertively follow my passion for writing and to carve out time for the things that are important to me.

Although I can't say that I am better off for having experienced the past two years, I feel that I have made the most of the situation and encourage you to try and do the same when life tosses obstacles in your way. Unfortunate accidents, illnesses and pains have the ability to throw a shadow over your purpose in life, so it is up to you to create goals, gain control, and redefine what you want in moving forward. Take your time, but learn to accept your circumstance, and be assertive in attending to both your physical and mental health to ensure your own well-being for years to come. Life is a journey with plenty of opportunities to develop wisdom and depth of character, the process may not always be enjoyable, but you would be surprised how much a positive attitude can steer your ship in the right direction.

# Take Aways and Resources

## Take Aways

→ Good posture involves using your rib cage to support your shoulders, not your shoulders to support your rib cage.

→ Moms are amazing and should be treated as such.

→ Women, whether they are in pain or not, should work with a physiotherapist postpartum to help return their bodies to "normal."

→ Even if you have lost touch with your body for years, you can rediscover it with some guidance.

→ Standing, walking, sitting, and breathing well are learned life skills and can be improved.

→ Learn from everything that life throws your way and never give up. Never.

## Website

+ WhyThingsHurt.com: There are many more articles, videos, topics and discussion on my blog. Please use the comments section of my posts to reach out to me with questions, feedback and testimonials. Stories are a big part of pain and recovery.

# Conclusions

I hope that this book has helped you to build a context for how your body works on a physical and emotional level. It is my hope for you to understand that things happen in your body for a reason, and that it is more important to understand why than it is to put a name on a symptom. You should know that you are the only one who is looking out for your body and mind, and that the healthcare professionals around you can only do so much. You are what you do repeatedly, and you are a product of everything that you have done, seen and experienced up to this moment. It is important to acknowledge the lens through which you see the world in order to develop self-awareness, and recognize that what you are doing either helps or hinders your progress in life.

The healthcare industry is a huge, often dysfunctional machine that can easily chew you up and spit you out if you enter it as a passive bystander, but it can be amazingly effective if you determine how to gain control and awareness of what is happening to you. To avoid resentment or getting lost throughout the process, you should learn the basic roles and scopes of the professionals who you encounter, and educate yourself as much as possible so you can ask the right questions and advocate for yourself at every step of your journey. The squeaky wheel really does get the grease in medical systems, and the quiet, passive cogs can fall through the cracks. Try your best to be a critical thinker, and speak up if you have a question; healthcare professionals are busy people, but they will typically try their best to help you understand what is going on.

Doctors do amazing things. They are great at keeping people alive, but they are not always your best source of advice when it comes to pain, health, or general well-being. Having a good doctor on your team is an invaluable asset, but you should realize that other health professionals may possess a much broader set of skills and experience than your physician in dealing with your problems. To maximize your health, your best course of action is to surround yourself with a variety of health professionals with overlapping, yet different knowledge bases to provide you with options and to allow you to critically analyze the advice you receive. Doctors are intelligent people, but they tend to rely on pills, surgeries, and diagnostic tests that are a parallel universe to health and well-being. Allied health professionals like physiotherapists, massage therapists, chiropractors, and naturopaths all play an important role in your quality of life, and you should strive to build a team of people who work for you, without putting blind faith in any one person.

Our bodies react to the forces we put them through, and our minds try to make sense of our experiences. These two concepts of our physical and mental states are weaved together in more ways than we can imagine, and unfortunately, the conventional healthcare system is usually unable to address both in a proactive way. Evidence-based medicine is the concept in which physicians use the best-available research to guide their actions, which makes complete sense in principle, but in practice it can bias them away from more deeply learning about aspects of the human body that are more difficult to research with sound scientific rigor. Incredible surgeries and amazing medications fit the medical mantra of evidence, but paired with the requirement of compartmentalized specialty, I find that many doctors are blinded to what they don't know, because they already know so much.

The experience of completing my clinical Master's of Physical Therapy at McMaster University, a school known for its research practices, followed by mentorship and experience working with world-respected health gurus, has biased me to focusing on clinical mastery over evidence-based practice. When working in a field that is considered a conservative intervention like physical therapy, I value the wisdom of the few who have interacted with other humans in a physical way for thirty to forty years more than I value the randomized controlled studies that generate vague, guiding statements of practice.

I have had the opportunities to work closely with physiotherapist Diane Lee, train under pain guru Dr. Chan Gunn, and be mentored by therapists directly connected with osteopath Jean-Pierre Barral. Diane helped me see the bigger picture when working with clients through her Integrated Systems Model. Dr. Gunn gave me the most powerful tool to help clients with IMS dry needling, and the Barral Institute helped me to access anatomy with my hands in an entirely new way. The experience of working with my clients as part of their journeys, as well as my own, has earned me an honorary degree in counseling psychology that I refer to as Why Things Hurt.

My experiences have taught me that perspective and attitude are the most important things to keep in check through the good times and the bad. I have learned that whining gets you nowhere and only annoys everyone around you. I have created a need to manage my own space and to understand the value of addressing my past in helping to control my future. Life has become busy for me these past ten years, but I offer you this book as proof that, as long as you find a way to keep moving in the right direction, you will eventually end up where you want to be. My kids, wife, mortgage, business, injuries, and life all could have stopped me from pursuing my goal of becoming an author, but I accepted my roles and responsibilities and kept nudging forward over the years, and my persistence and perseverance are paying off.

Please use this book as an opportunity to take a constructive look at yourself and how you approach preventative health going forward. Help educate others about how their bodies work and be assertive in your interactions with your healthcare system. Know that, while your body slowly degenerates over time, it doesn't have to directly correlate with pain, and that even though your doctor may not understand them, IMS and manual therapy are invaluable tools to help your body function. Remember that you were not born wearing shoes, and that your feet may hold some answers to your pain and posture if you let them out from time to time. Lastly, respect your mother, but now it's your turn to teach her how to stand up straight!

# Acknowledgments

Thank you to my parents for teaching me the value of play and an appreciation of the human body.

Thank you to my wife for putting up with all my ideas, supporting me, challenging me, caring for me and loving me.

Thank you to my kids for being my outlet and motivation to keep moving forward.

Thank you to my mentors and influencers for guiding me, teaching me and giving me shoulders to stand on: Diane Lee, Dr. Chan Gunn, Annabel MacKenzie, Judy Russel, Ron Mariotti, JP Barral, Shirley Sahrmann, and Braeden Lalor.

Thank you to my business partner and friend Harry Toor for complementing my skill set, being a sounding board, always having a great attitude and positive energy.

Thank you to all the staff at Envision Physiotherapy, Essential Kinetics, The Movement Studio and Kor Manual Therapy for working and learning together so effectively. I am better by being surrounded by all of you every day.

Thank you to all my clients for letting me into your lives over the past thirteen years. I have learned a little something from all of you!

Thank you to the countless surgeons and nurses that tried to put my eye back together: Dr. Ma, Dr. Maberley, Dr. Schendel, Dr. Faber, Dr. Lyons, and Dr. Rossman.

Thank you to all my friends and family that have supported me through my journey. You are a part of me and I wouldn't be here without you.

CPSIA information can be obtained
at www.ICGtesting.com
Printed in the USA
BVHW04s0221140618
519036BV00018B/177/P

9 780995 324107